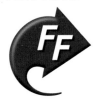

Fast Facts

F035764

F

CW01096257

WITHDRAWN

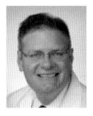

Thomas Mahl MD
Clinical Professor, Gastroenterology
Department of Medicine
University at Buffalo School of Medicine
Buffalo, New York, USA

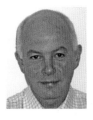

John O'Grady MD
Consultant Hepatologist
Institute of Liver Studies
King's College School of Medicine
London, UK

Declaration of Independence
This book is as balanced and as practical as we can make it.
Ideas for improvement are always welcome: feedback@fastfacts.com

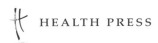

HEALTH PRESS

Fast Facts: Liver Disorders
First edition 2006
Second edition November 2014

Text © 2014 Thomas Mahl, John O'Grady
© 2014 in this edition Health Press Limited
Health Press Limited, Elizabeth House, Queen Street, Abingdon,
Oxford OX14 3LN, UK
Tel: +44 (0)1235 523233

Book orders can be placed by telephone or via the website. For regional distributors
or to order via the website, please go to: fastfacts.com

For telephone orders, please call +44 (0)1752 202301 (UK, Europe and Asia–
Pacific), 1 800 247 6553 (USA, toll free) or +1 419 281 1802 (Americas).

Fast Facts is a trademark of Health Press Limited.

A CIP record for this title is available from the British Library.

ISBN 978-1-908541-64-2

Mahl T (Thomas)
Fast Facts: Liver Disorders/
Thomas Mahl, John O'Grady

Medical illustrations by Dee McLean, London, and
Annamaria Dutto, Withernsea, UK.
Typesetting and page layout by Zed, Oxford, UK.
Printed by Latimer Trend and Company, Plymouth, UK.

Text printed on biodegradable and recyclable paper
manufactured using elemental chlorine free (ECF)
wood pulp from well-managed forests.

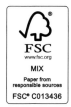

FSC
www.fsc.org
MIX
Paper from
responsible sources
FSC® C013436

List of abbreviations

AFP: alpha fetoprotein

AIH: autoimmune hepatitis

ALD: alcoholic liver disease

ALT: alanine aminotransferase

AMA: antimitochondrial antibodies

AST: aspartate aminotransferase

ATD: α_1 antitrypsin deficiency

BMI: body mass index

CT: computed tomography

DILI: drug-induced liver injury

ES: endoscopic sclerotherapy

EVL: endoscopic variceal ligation

GGT: gamma-glutamyltransferase

HBeAg/Ab: hepatitis B 'e' antigen/antibody

HBsAg/Ab: hepatitis B 'surface' antigen/antibody

HBV: hepatitis B virus

HCC: hepatocellular carcinoma

HCV: hepatitis C virus

HELLP: hemolysis, elevated liver enzymes, low platelet count

Ig: immunoglobulin

INR: international normalized ratio

LDLT: living donor liver transplant

LVP: large-volume paracentesis

MELD: model for end-stage liver disease

NAFLD: non-alcoholic fatty liver disease

NASH: non-alcoholic steatohepatitis

5NT: 5'nucleotidase

pANCA: perinuclear antineutrophil cytoplasmic antibody

PBC: primary biliary cirrhosis

PCR: polymerase chain reaction

PELD: pediatric end-stage liver disease

PiZZ: protease inhibitor, Z variant, homozygous (a mutation of the α1 antitrypsin gene)

PSC: primary sclerosing cholangitis

PT: prothrombin time

PTLD: post-transplant lymphoproliferative disease

SAAG: serum–ascites albumin gradient

SBP: spontaneous bacterial peritonitis

TACE: transarterial chemoembolization

TIPS: transjugular intrahepatic portosystemic shunt

TNF: tumor necrosis factor

UDCA: ursodeoxycholic acid

Introduction

Our aim in this book is to provide a succinct and practical guide to the diagnosis and therapeutic management of liver disease.

Given the frequent presentation of liver disorders in general practice, accurate diagnosis and an understanding of the indicators of severe disease are essential in order to swiftly identify the small cohort in need of referral for specialist treatment. This book is designed to provide an organized approach to isolating the origin of the disorder, correcting the cause, minimizing permanent damage and risk, and monitoring and managing recovery.

Since the first edition of *Fast Facts: Liver Disorders* there have been significant improvements in the treatment of hepatitis B and C, new understandings of the pathogenesis of hemochromatosis and a significant increase in liver cancers.

Alcoholic liver disease remains the major cause of liver disease in Western countries and there is an emerging epidemic of similar non-alcoholic liver disease related to obesity and the metabolic syndrome. Our review of these chronic disorders is pitched at understanding the most important issues as quickly as possible. With increasing numbers of patients undergoing liver function tests and ultrasonic evaluation of the liver, quick access to a commonsense approach to investigation and simple explanations are of huge benefit. In addition, many non-specialists and primary care providers are encountering patients who have been recipients of liver transplants. We deal with some of the more common clinical problems associated with the procedure, which may require attention in the community.

The field of liver disease has recently entered a happy time. Hepatology used to be just a diagnostic sport with few effective treatments for liver disease. That has changed – and will change further in the next few years. We believe that the format of this handbook will be of practical use to all members of the primary care team, junior doctors and nurse specialists; indeed, all who require instant access to the key facts on liver disorders.

1 Investigating liver disease

Liver disorders are encountered frequently in general practice. In the UK, while mortality rates from other major causes of disease are falling, mortality from liver disease continues to increase, and accounts for approximately 2% of all deaths in England. In the USA, recent data suggest that 5.5 million people have chronic liver disease. Many asymptomatic patients will have elevated liver test results, although the incidence varies considerably between populations with differing risk profiles. The goals of the physician's investigation are to understand the origin of the liver injury, to correct its cause and to prevent permanent organ dysfunction (i.e. cirrhosis). An organized approach to investigating liver abnormalities allows the physician to reach conclusions promptly, and avoids excessive cost or risk to the patient.

Liver anatomy and physiology

The liver is uniquely positioned between the gut and the systemic circulation to receive blood rich in both nutrients and toxins; it facilitates the metabolism of nutrients and destroys toxins. Blood travelling to the spleen, stomach, pancreas, gallbladder and intestines is collected in the hepatic portal vein and delivered to the tissues of the liver where it is processed. Blood leaves the tissues of the liver via the hepatic veins. The liver also has its own system of arteries and arterioles that provide oxygenated blood to its tissues (Figure 1.1).

The liver is protected by the right lower ribs, so usually only a few centimeters can be felt on physical examination. It is often enlarged in the initial stages of disease, and its firmness will provide the examiner with a rough idea of the degree of fibrosis. In later disease stages, the liver may shrink and regress under the ribs, making it difficult or impossible to feel.

Hepatocytes perform most of the liver's functions, including bile production. The bile drains into bile canaliculi (microscopic canals), which join together into larger intrahepatic bile ducts. These in turn join the larger left and right hepatic ducts, which unite to form the common hepatic duct. The common hepatic duct joins the cystic duct

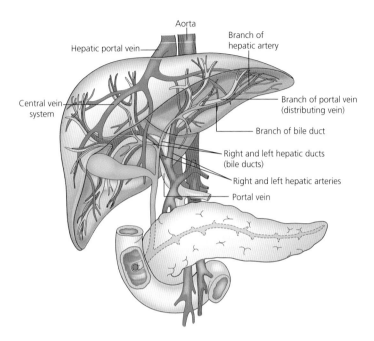

Figure 1.1 Anatomy of the liver, depicting the blood supply and structure of the biliary tree (intra- and extrahepatic bile ducts).

from the gallbladder to form the common bile duct, which courses posteriorly to the duodenum and pancreas.

This network of various sized ducts branching through the liver is known as the biliary tree, and is an important exit from the liver for organic anions, bilirubin, cholesterol and a host of other products. The external biliary tree travels through crowded territory – over the hepatic artery and portal vein, under the duodenum and then through the pancreas. Malignancy of the pancreas often presents with biliary obstruction.

Acute liver injuries

Acute liver injuries are defined by hepatologists as those that resolve within 6 months. Patients with acute liver disease typically have no previous history of liver injury. They may complain of fatigue, anorexia, malaise and discomfort in the right upper quadrant of the abdomen. Jaundice may be seen and tender hepatomegaly elicited. Significant pain and fever suggest biliary obstruction.

Acute liver injuries (e.g. viral hepatitis, exposure to a toxin or medication) typically resolve once the offending agent is removed or the viral infection resolves, and usually there are no sequelae. Occasionally, however, liver injury is so severe that the patient does not have enough hepatocytes remaining to allow for homeostasis – a condition called fulminant hepatic failure or acute liver failure (see page 24).

Chronic liver injuries

The primary care provider more often encounters chronic, rather than acute, liver disease. Patients typically present with few symptoms, and diagnosis is on the basis of abnormal blood results on routine examination. They may complain of fatigue and malaise. The examiner may find stigmata of chronic liver disease, such as gynecomastia, spider nevi, telangiectasia and palmar erythema. The liver is usually enlarged and may be firm; a tender liver is uncommon. If advanced liver disease has developed (e.g. cirrhosis), signs of portal hypertension such as splenomegaly or ascites may be present.

History

As with all medical conditions, it is vital to obtain a thorough and accurate history (Table 1.1).

History of jaundice should be determined with respect to liver disease. Risk factors for viral hepatitis include prior transfusion, multiple sexual partners, tattoo application and needle sharing.

Alcohol intake. Alcohol, of course, is a common hepatic toxin, and physicians must be adept at determining a patient's alcohol consumption. Unfortunately, this is significantly more difficult to accomplish in practice than in theory. Alcoholism is a disease of denial, and many patients will not admit to, or even realize, how much alcohol they consume. A simple tool such as a standard drinks measure, or a visual guide to units (Figure 1.2), will assist health professionals in tackling the subject of excessive alcohol consumption

TABLE 1.1

Areas to cover in a history for liver disorders

- Clinical history, including previous:
  - jaundice
  - blood transfusion
- Social history, including:
  - alcohol intake
  - tattoos
  - needle sharing
  - multiple sexual partners
- Family history of liver disease
- Occupational history to reveal exposure to toxins
- Current medications

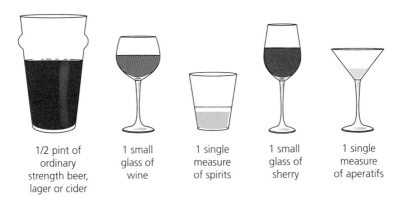

| 1/2 pint of ordinary strength beer, lager or cider | 1 small glass of wine | 1 single measure of spirits | 1 small glass of sherry | 1 single measure of aperatifs |

Figure 1.2 A visual guide to 'one unit' of alcohol in standard drinks.

with their patients in a sensitive but realistic way. Short validated questionnaires, such as the Alcohol Use Disorders Identification Test (AUDIT), developed by the World Health Organization (WHO), or the CAGE questionnaire are available online (see Useful resources). The simplified AUDIT-C test, which comprises just three questions, is particularly useful if time is short (Table 1.2).

TABLE 1.2

Validated questionnaires for determining hazardous alcohol consumption

AUDIT-C

How often do you have a drink containing alcohol?

a. Never
b. Monthly or less
c. 2–4 times a month
d. 2–3 times a week
e. 4 or more times a week

How many standard drinks containing alcohol do you have on a typical day?

a. 1 or 2
b. 3 or 4
c. 5 or 6
d. 7 to 9
e. 10 or more

How often do you have six or more drinks on one occasion?

a. Never
b. Less than monthly
c. Monthly
d. Weekly
e. Daily or almost daily

a=0; b=1; c=2; d=3; e=4

Positive result – hazardous drinking or active alcohol use disorder

≥ 4 in men, ≥ 3 in women

However, when all points are from Question 1 alone (questions 2 and 3 are zero), it can be assumed the patient is drinking below recommended levels; review the patient's alcohol intake over the past few months to confirm accuracy.

CAGE

1. Have you ever felt you needed to **C**ut down on your drinking?

2. Have people **A**nnoyed you by criticizing your drinking?

3. Have you ever felt **G**uilty about drinking?

4. Have you ever felt you needed a drink first thing in the morning (**E**ye-opener) to steady your nerves or to get rid of a hangover?

Two 'yes' responses indicate the need for further investigation.

Medications may also cause liver disease, so it is important to determine which medications a patient is taking, and particularly those temporally related to the development of the liver disorder. Some over-the-counter medications and herbal remedies have also been reported to cause liver abnormalities.

Occupational history. Although most hepatic toxins are no longer common in the workplace, an occupational history may reveal relevant exposures.

A family history of liver disease is equally important. In our experience the liver disease that most commonly clusters in a family is alcoholic liver disease (ALD), but other diseases such as Wilson's disease and hemochromatosis (see Chapter 6) should be considered.

Liver function tests

Liver enzymes. The liver typically responds to injury by releasing enzymes from hepatocytes and/or biliary epithelium. Elevated levels of enzymes of hepatocellular origin, such as aspartate aminotransferase (AST) and alanine aminotransferase (ALT), suggest injury to hepatocytes. Elevations in alkaline phosphatase suggest injury to the function or structure of the biliary system.

Aminotransferases (transaminases). AST is a mitochondrial enzyme found in the liver and other tissues, such as skeletal and myocardial muscle. ALT is a cytoplasmic enzyme found primarily in the liver. Both AST and ALT are released from injured hepatocytes, and elevated levels are found in the blood of patients with liver disease of diverse etiologies. In most liver disorders, ALT is higher than AST. When AST is higher than ALT (particularly if the ratio is greater than 2), ALD should be strongly suspected.

Elevations of aminotransferases do not necessarily correlate with the severity of liver injury. For example, in severe alcoholic hepatitis, aminotransferases may be no greater than four or five times the upper limit of normal, whereas in asymptomatic acute viral hepatitis, aminotransferase elevations can easily range from 20 to 100 times the upper limit of normal.

Alkaline phosphatase catalyzes phosphatase reactions in alkaline environments in vitro, but its function in vivo is not well defined. However, it has long been established that injury to the bile ducts, whether the extrahepatic bile ducts or the microscopic canaliculi that course through the liver, results in elevated alkaline phosphatase levels in the blood.

Alkaline phosphatase is not unique to the liver; it is also found in bone, and to a lesser extent in the placenta and intestine. Identifying which organ is releasing alkaline phosphatase is based on isoenzyme analysis. Patients with elevated alkaline phosphatase of hepatic origin usually have symptoms or signs of liver disease or other hepatic abnormalities on biochemical screening. In contrast, patients with elevated alkaline phosphatase of bone origin may complain of bone pain or may be diagnosed with Paget's disease or have a known malignancy. On occasion, however, elevated alkaline phosphatase is discovered as an isolated abnormality. In this case, further laboratory tests are required to determine its origin (Figure 1.3).

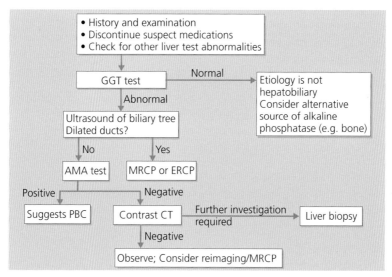

Figure 1.3 Investigational pathway to determine the origin of elevated alkaline phosphatase. AMA, antimitochondrial antibody; CT, computed tomography; ERCP, endoscopic retrograde cholangiopancreatography; GGT, gamma-glutamyltransferase; MRCP, magnetic resonance cholangiopancreatography; PBC, primary biliary cirrhosis.

The enzymes 5'nucleotidase (5NT) and gamma-glutamyltransferase (GGT) parallel alkaline phosphatase of hepatic origin. Thus, in liver disease, 5NT and GGT will be elevated as well as the alkaline phosphatase, whereas in bone disease 5NT and GGT levels will be normal. GGT levels can also be useful in the diagnosis of ALD, as GGT is rapidly inducible by alcohol and often reaches impressive elevations in patients with even mild alcoholic liver injury.

As with the aminotransferases, alkaline phosphatase levels do not necessarily correlate with the severity of liver injury or dysfunction. Prothrombin time (PT) and albumin and bilirubin levels are better measures of liver function.

Prothrombin time. Most clotting factors are produced by the liver. Thus, measurement of PT is a reliable marker of liver function. Because the clotting proteins require vitamin K as a cofactor, vitamin K deficiency must be ruled out as a cause of an increased PT. Parenteral administration of vitamin K to patients with vitamin K deficiency usually corrects the PT within 12–24 hours, whereas vitamin K has a negligible effect in liver failure. Occasionally, vitamin K deficiency and liver disease coincide. With cholestatic liver disorders, such as primary biliary cirrhosis and primary sclerosing cholangitis, the absorption of fat-soluble vitamins such as vitamin K can be impaired. Thus, administering vitamin K to a patient with an elevated PT is reasonable. However, repeated daily injections of vitamin K when there is no apparent improvement in PT are not helpful.

Albumin is a protein synthesized only in the liver. Thus, measurement of the albumin concentration is a reasonable test of the synthetic capacity of the liver. It should be noted, however, that albumin lost through the urine (e.g. nephrotic syndrome) or through the gastrointestinal tract (e.g. inflammatory bowel disease) could mimic hypoalbuminemia of liver origin. Similarly, a patient who is malnourished may not deliver enough substrate to the liver for adequate synthesis of albumin. Malnutrition and liver disease frequently coexist.

Bilirubin. Measurement of the serum bilirubin concentration is perhaps the most important test of liver function. Bilirubin is a product of the turnover of red blood cells, with a relatively constant value in the serum. Hyperbilirubinemia signifies one of several scenarios.

- An increased load of bilirubin may be delivered to the liver from the periphery, as occurs in hemolysis, and the resulting hyperbilirubinemia is predominantly of the unconjugated fraction. Review of the peripheral smear or measurement of lactate dehydrogenase or haptoglobin helps to identify hemolysis as a cause of increased bilirubin levels.
- Injury of liver cells (e.g. in hepatitis or cirrhosis) is another cause of elevated bilirubin levels. Both acute and chronic liver disease may result in hyperbilirubinemia that is usually predominantly of the conjugated fraction.
- Obstruction to bile flow, which can occur anywhere along the biliary tree from the microscopic canaliculi to the large extrahepatic bile ducts, can also lead to elevated serum bilirubin. Obstruction may result from physical abnormalities, such as a stone resting in the common bile duct or a tumor in the pancreas, that physically prevent bilirubin from exiting the liver. More subtle insults can also occur, such as injuries to the microscopic biliary canaliculi by medications such as estrogen and ampicillin/clavulanic acid.
- Sepsis may cause dysfunction of the mechanism of bilirubin transport across the canalicular membrane, leading to hyperbilirubinemia.
- Inherited disorders of bilirubin metabolism may result in increased serum bilirubin levels. Gilbert's syndrome is the most common of these, affecting at least 4% of the population. Gilbert's syndrome results from a mutation in the gene that controls the production of uridine diphosphate glucuronosyltransferase, the enzyme that conjugates bilirubin from its water-insoluble to its water-soluble form. Thus, these patients have elevations of unconjugated (indirect) bilirubin levels. An important clue to the diagnosis of Gilbert's syndrome is otherwise normal liver function, i.e. normal albumin concentration, PT, aminotransferases and alkaline phosphatase levels. These patients only require reassurance.

Imaging and biopsy

Radiology plays an important role in the evaluation of patients with some forms of liver disease.

Ultrasonography is particularly useful for examining the hepatic parenchyma for abnormalities (e.g. tumors or other space-occupying lesions) and the biliary tree for dilation induced by distal obstruction. Increased echo texture is usually interpreted as a sign of fatty infiltration of the liver or hepatocellular inflammation, such as that which accompanies viral hepatitis. It is our opinion, however, that this is neither sensitive nor specific, and findings must be interpreted in the overall clinical context.

Computed tomography (CT) can identify space-occupying lesions measuring more than 1 cm. In addition, fatty infiltration of the liver can be diagnosed with reasonable sensitivity and specificity. CT also provides good views of the biliary tree, pancreas and other intra-abdominal organs.

Biopsy. A liver biopsy is the gold standard for evaluation of liver disease. Although patients approach biopsy with trepidation, it is safe and quite simple to perform. Most liver biopsies are now performed under ultrasound guidance on an outpatient basis. Generally, a biopsy is safe provided that the PT is prolonged by no more than a few seconds and the platelet count is greater than $70\,000 \times 10^{-6}$/L. A liver biopsy usually allows a definitive diagnosis of the underlying liver disorder and staging of the disease (severity of permanent liver injury; fibrosis; cirrhosis).

Elastography is a non-invasive method of estimating the extent of liver fibrosis, which is now becoming more widely used. It replaces the need for a liver biopsy for that indication and is particularly utilized in patients with hepatitis C.

Investigational pathways for mildly abnormal liver function tests

Mild elevations in AST, ALT and GGT are commonly detected on programmed health evaluations or during the investigation of unrelated symptoms. An elevated GGT level is particularly common, with levels up to five times the upper limit of normal, usually with a lesser degree of abnormality in alkaline phosphatase. The serum aminotransferases (transaminases) may be normal or increased to four to five times the upper limit of normal. Assuming, for this example, that the serum bilirubin, albumin and PT are normal, initial steps are to:

- consider a repeat of the tests to eliminate laboratory error
- take a history of alcohol usage
- elicit drug exposure during the previous 6 months
- screen for diabetes mellitus or family history of diabetes
- weigh, and calculate body mass index (BMI).

Alcoholic liver disease. Regular alcohol use can account for this pattern of abnormal liver function tests, even if the intake is not considered excessive. This particularly applies to women. An AST level that is higher than the ALT level supports alcohol as the cause. Elevated mean corpuscular volume provides strong supporting evidence that alcohol is the underlying cause. A trial of abstinence from alcohol for 3 months will determine the contribution of alcohol to the abnormality (an algorithm for investigations is shown in Figure 1.4).

Non-alcoholic fatty liver disease is another explanation for this pattern of abnormal liver function tests. This diagnosis is more likely against the background of:

- credible history of minimal or no alcohol consumption
- increased BMI or obesity
- non-insulin-dependent diabetes or family history of diabetes
- hyperlipidemia, particularly hypertriglyceridemia.

An ultrasound examination will detect fatty infiltration in many cases, but its absence does not exclude the possible diagnosis of fatty liver.

The liver function profile may underestimate the severity of the liver disease in a minority of patients. A liver biopsy should be performed if there are any indicators of portal hypertension (e.g. platelet count below normal or an enlarged spleen on ultrasonography).

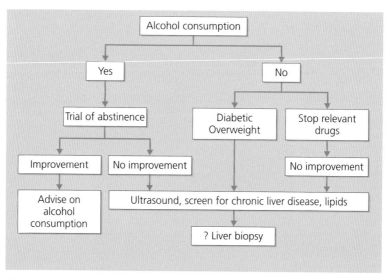

Figure 1.4 Investigational pathway for mild elevations in aspartate aminotransferase, alanine aminotransferase and gamma-glutamyltransferase.

Isolated increase in aminotransferases. Serum aminotransferases may be mildly increased in association with a range of innocuous intercurrent infections. A solitary finding does not warrant immediate extensive investigation (Figure 1.5) unless a risk factor for chronic viral hepatitis is identified (Table 1.3).

In other instances, liver function tests should be repeated after about 3 months and investigations performed if the abnormality persists. Screening for chronic viral hepatitis B and C is the most critical part of the evaluation. When the viral screen is negative, investigations should be extended to cover other causes of chronic liver disease. These include:

- autoantibody screen
- immunoglobulin measurements
- ceruloplasmin measurement – particularly in those under 40 years
- ferritin measurement
- determination of α_1 antitrypsin phenotype.

An ultrasound scan of the liver and possibly a liver biopsy complete the investigation in most instances.

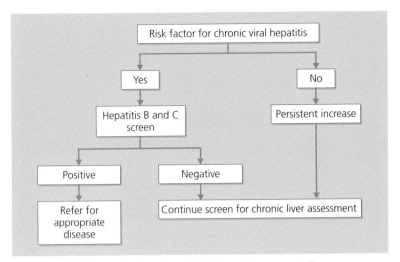

Figure 1.5 Investigational pathway for isolated increases in liver aminotransferases.

TABLE 1.3

Risk factors for chronic viral hepatitis

- Ethnic background associated with high risk
- Needle sharing at any period of life
- Receipt of blood products before 1990
- Tattoos
- Men who have sex with men, or known risky sexual exposure

Isolated increase in serum bilirubin. If this is the only abnormality in the liver function profile, it is usually due to Gilbert's syndrome, a congenital abnormality that occurs in 4% of the population (see page 15). The bilirubin is predominantly unconjugated. The main differential diagnosis is chronic hemolytic anemia (e.g. due to spherocytosis). The bilirubin increases during intercurrent illnesses and, as a result, the patient may inappropriately attribute the associated symptoms to being jaundiced. Gilbert's syndrome is entirely innocuous.

Key points – investigating liver disease

- Elevated levels of aspartate aminotransferase and alanine aminotransferase suggest injury to hepatocytes.
- An elevated level of alkaline phosphatase suggests injury to structures of the biliary tree.
- Prothrombin time (after vitamin K) and serum albumin are used to assess the liver's ability to synthesize proteins.
- Increases in serum bilirubin occur for many reasons, but generally indicate severe disease.
- A liver biopsy is the gold standard for evaluation of liver disease.

Key references

Addley J, Mitchell RM. Advances in the investigation of obstructive jaundice. *Curr Gastroenterol Rep* 2012;14:511–19.

Coates P. Liver function tests. *Aust Fam Physician* 2011;40:113–15.

Lalani T, Couto CA, Rosen MP et al. ACR appropriateness criteria jaundice. *J Am Coll Radiol* 2013;10:402–9.

National End of Life Care Intelligence Network. *Deaths from liver disease. Implications for end of life care in England.* Bristol: South West Public Health Observatory, 2012.

Pratt DS, Kaplan MM. Evaluation of abnormal liver-enzyme results in asymptomatic patients. *N Engl J Med* 2000;342:1266–71.

Rockey DC, Caldwell SH, Goodman ZD et al. AASLD Position Paper – Liver Biopsy. *Hepatology* 2009;49:1017–44.

Strassburg CP. Hyperbilirubinemia syndromes (Gilbert-Meulengracht, Crigler-Najjar, Dubin-Johnson, and Rotor syndrome). *Best Pract Res Clin Gastroenterol* 2010;24:555–71.

Winger J, Michefelder A. Diagnostic approach to the patient with jaundice. *Prim Care* 2011;38:469–82.

Acute liver disease refers to diseases of less than 6 months' duration at the time of presentation. This category of disease excludes first presentations of cirrhosis, with a few exceptions, such as when hepatitis B or Wilson's disease present with the syndrome of acute liver failure. There are three major categories of acute liver disease:
- hepatitis
- cholestasis
- vascular disease.

The associated symptoms and biochemical profiles differentiate between these patterns of disease (Table 2.1). Jaundice is the typical

TABLE 2.1

Characteristics of the main presentations of acute liver disease

	Hepatitis	Cholestasis	Vascular
Jaundice	Common	Common	Mild
Dark urine	Yes	Yes	No
Pale feces	Unusual	Yes	No
Itch	Unusual	Yes	No
Ascites	Unusual	No	Yes
Serum bilirubin	Variable but may be high	Variable but may be high	< 100 µmol/L (< 6 mg/dL)
Aminotransferases	> 500 IU/L but often much higher	< 300 IU/L	Usually < 300 IU/L
Cholestatic enzymes	Usually < 3 × normal	High	Usually < 2 × normal
Albumin	Normal	Normal	Normal or low
Significance of coagulopathy	Risk of acute liver failure	Vitamin K deficiency	Risk of acute liver failure

presentation of both hepatitis and cholestasis; the sudden onset of ascites is the most common presentation of vascular disease.

Hepatitis

Viral infections and drug reactions account for most cases of acute hepatitis with an identifiable cause (Table 2.2). The liver function profile reveals a predominant increase in the serum aminotransferases (transaminases), with figures in excess of 1000 IU/L in the early phase. The serum bilirubin level increases as the aminotransferase levels fall. The severity of the acute hepatitis is reflected in three clinical categories:

- uncomplicated hepatitis
- severe hepatitis
- acute liver failure.

The development of a coagulopathy (prolonged prothrombin time [PT] or international normalized ratio [INR], reduced factor V levels)

TABLE 2.2

Causes of acute hepatitis

Viral	Drugs
• Hepatitis A	• Dose-dependent: paracetamol (acetaminophen)
• Hepatitis B (occasionally with hepatitis D)	• Idiosyncratic (e.g. isoniazid, amiodarone, phenytoin, non-steroidal anti-inflammatory drugs, Ecstacy)
• Hepatitis E	
• Seronegative or indeterminate hepatitis	
• Leptospirosis (Weil's disease)	**Other causes**
• Rare	• Autoimmune hepatitis
– hepatitis C	• Ischemia
– herpes simplex	
– cytomegalovirus	
– Epstein–Barr virus	
– adenovirus	

determines the transition to severe hepatitis. The onset of acute liver failure is signaled by the onset of encephalopathy (a neurological syndrome ranging in severity from drowsiness and poor concentration to coma).

Acute hepatitis has a prodromal phase, during which anorexia, nausea, vomiting and loss of appetite for food and cigarettes are typical features. The prodromal phase is as short as 1 week for hepatitis A but may be as long as 3 months for hepatitis B. This is usually followed by the onset of jaundice, although this is not always the case in young children. The prodromal symptoms characteristically improve once jaundice develops. The jaundice resolves over variable periods but usually within 6 weeks of onset. Lethargy may be profound and persist for months after the jaundice has cleared.

Hepatitis A is contracted by the orofecal route. Childhood exposure is now the norm only in developing countries; accordingly, in the Western world, immunity levels in teenagers have fallen to below 5%. Childhood infection usually causes a non-specific illness; the likelihood of developing jaundice increases with age at acquisition. Adults may acquire hepatitis from infected water or shellfish, travel to endemic areas or occupational or sexual exposure.

Hepatitis A is one of the few causes of acute hepatitis that results in fever. The risk of developing acute liver failure is only 0.1% overall, increasing exponentially with age. Hepatitis is a biphasic illness in 6–10% of cases and is followed by a cholestatic phase in about 5%.

There is no specific treatment for hepatitis A, and it does not have a chronic carrier state in humans. Vaccination against hepatitis A is effective and is advised for travelers to endemic areas, individuals at occupational risk, patients with chronic liver disease and men who have sex with men.

Hepatitis B is contracted by vertical transmission, sexual exposure and contact with infected blood. Vertical transmission occurs at birth and is the main route of infection in highly endemic areas. Chronic carriage follows neonatal exposure in 95% of cases, whereas only 5% of adults who contract hepatitis B become chronic carriers.

An increasing number of antiviral agents have become available for the treatment of patients with acute hepatitis B. Vaccination is effective in preventing infection in over 95% of individuals. Target populations for vaccination include healthcare workers and men who have sex with men.

Seronegative or indeterminate hepatitis are two of the terms used to describe a presumed viral hepatitis for which no cause can be identified. This entity occurs particularly in patients developing acute liver failure. Although assumed to be viral, this condition has a propensity for middle-aged women and does not occur in clusters. Unrecognized toxins or autoimmune processes are alternative explanations.

Hepatitis C and E. Hepatitis C is rarely identified as a cause of acute hepatitis. Hepatitis E is common in the Indian subcontinent, and there has been an increase in sporadic cases identified in the West. The natural history is similar to that of hepatitis A. However, hepatitis E is associated with a peculiarly high mortality in pregnant women. There is no effective vaccine for hepatitis C or hepatitis E.

Leptospirosis or Weil's disease is an unusual cause of acute hepatitis, typically acquired by contact with rat's urine. Rapid diagnosis is important because of the potential for effective treatment with penicillin in the early phase. Characteristic features include fever, hemorrhagic skin rash and renal dysfunction.

Other causes. Idiosyncratic reactions leading to hepatitis may follow exposure to a wide range of drugs; some of the more common causes are listed in Table 2.2.

Autoimmune hepatitis may present for the first time with an episode of florid hepatitis.

Acute liver failure

Acute liver failure is a life-threatening complication of acute hepatitis and a number of other liver diseases (Wilson's disease, acute fatty liver of pregnancy, Budd–Chiari syndrome and *Amanita phalloides* mushroom poisoning). The definition of acute liver failure is based on the development of encephalopathy within 12 weeks of the onset of jaundice. Hypoglycemia may mimic encephalopathy, but its occurrence is an independent indicator of severe liver injury and risk of later progression to encephalopathy. A coagulopathy is invariably present. PT rises and the bilirubin rockets upwards. Many of these patients will die unless they receive a liver transplant.

Acute liver failure causes multisystem failure (Figure 2.1). Neurological complications are a major cause of death, as a result of either severe cerebral hypoxia or brainstem herniation complicating cerebral edema. Sepsis and circulatory failure account for most other deaths. The development of renal failure also indicates a poorer prognosis. Overall, about 30% of patients survive without surgery, 40% undergo emergency liver transplantation with survival rates of up to 80%, and the remaining 30% die. Specific prognostic models are used in specialist centers to determine prognosis and the need for liver transplantation. Outcome is heavily influenced by the underlying etiology, the age of the patient and the rate of progression of the disease. A number of easily recognizable scenarios that are associated with either a favorable or unfavorable outcome are given in Table 2.3.

Paracetamol (acetaminophen) overdose induces a distinct pattern of acute liver failure. Acidosis may be an early feature, and failure to reverse the acidosis within 24 hours of drug ingestion is associated with a very high mortality. Patients at risk of acute liver failure are identified by the development of a coagulopathy, and encephalopathy typically develops on the third or fourth day after the overdose. Renal failure is more common and earlier than with other causes of acute liver failure. Progression to acute liver failure is usually prevented by the administration of N-acetylcysteine within 16–24 hours of the overdose. Later administration of N-acetylcysteine may also modify the severity of the disease.

Wilson's disease, an inherited disorder of copper metabolism, may present with many of the clinical features of acute liver failure. It is

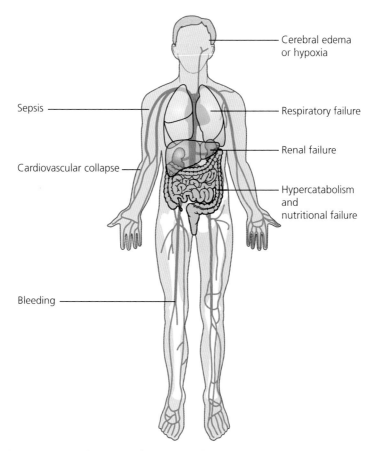

Figure 2.1 Complications of acute liver failure, leading to multisystem failure.

therefore classified as acute, even though the majority of patients have cirrhosis at the time of presentation. Hemolytic anemia and ascites early in the course of the disease are characteristics of Wilson's disease.

Cholestasis

Cholestatic jaundice is characterized predominantly by elevations in alkaline phosphatase and gamma-glutamyltransferase (GGT).

Extrahepatic biliary obstruction is the cause of most cases of cholestasis (Table 2.4). The presence of pain points to gallstone

TABLE 2.3

Features suggestive of a favorable or unfavorable outcome in acute liver failure

Favorable

- Paracetamol (acetaminophen) overdose with no evidence of metabolic acidosis or renal failure, despite the presence of a severe coagulopathy
- Pregnancy-related syndromes
- Viral hepatitis A or B, encephalopathy developing within 7 days of onset of jaundice

Unfavorable

- Seronegative hepatitis or idiosyncratic drug reactions
- Wilson's disease
- Encephalopathy developing more than 7 days after onset of jaundice
- Jaundice for more than 4 weeks despite coagulopathy and encephalopathy being mild
- Young children
- Adults over 40 years of age
- Paracetamol overdose with severe metabolic acidosis or combination of severe encephalopathy, renal failure and severe coagulopathy

disease; conversely, the absence of pain suggests malignant disease, especially in older patients. Biliary obstruction causes dilation of the bile ducts and is easily detected on ultrasound examination, which is the initial screening procedure. More precise definition of the site of the obstruction is then obtained by endoscopic or magnetic resonance cholangiography.

Intrahepatic causes of cholestasis should be considered when there is no evidence of duct dilation on ultrasound examination. The dominant clinical features are jaundice and pruritus. Other features

TABLE 2.4

Causes of extrahepatic biliary obstruction

- Gallstones
- Cholangiocarcinoma
  - hilar
  - mid or lower bile duct
- Ampullary adenocarcinoma
- Adenocarcinoma of the head of the pancreas
- Benign inflammatory stricture
- Postsurgical stricture (particularly after laparoscopic cholecystectomy)
- Primary sclerosing cholangitis, with or without complicating cholangiocarcinoma

include dark urine and pale stools, and weight loss may be considerable. The liver function profile comprises elevated serum bilirubin, serum alkaline phosphatase and GGT but no features that distinguish intrahepatic from extrahepatic biliary obstruction. There may be an abnormality in coagulation tests in protracted cases, but this is corrected rapidly by parenteral administration of vitamin K. There is no specific therapy other than symptomatic relief, particularly of the pruritus – colestyramine (cholestyramine), ursodeoxycholic acid, rifampicin (rifampin). The duration of the cholestatic episode is variable but it can last for many months.

Idiosyncratic drug reaction is another cause of cholestasis (Table 2.5). Drug-induced cholestasis is likely to recur with repeated exposure to the offending agent. Cholestasis induced by estrogen in contraceptive pills indicates a high risk of developing cholestasis during subsequent pregnancies.

Benign recurrent cholestasis is a poorly understood entity of recurring episodes of cholestasis without an obvious precipitating cause.

TABLE 2.5

Drugs associated with cholestatic reactions

• Estrogens and androgens	• Amitriptyline
• Chlorpromazine	• Carbamazepine
• Tricyclic antidepressants	• Erythromycin
• Barbiturates	• Flucloxacillin
• Phenytoin	

Other causes of cholestasis include injury to small bile ducts (e.g. as a manifestation of flucloxacillin hepatotoxicity). Cholestasis may herald Hodgkin's lymphoma as a paraneoplastic syndrome.

Vascular disease

Hepatic vein thrombosis, or Budd–Chiari syndrome, may have an acute presentation with abdominal pain and massive ascites. The liver function profile shows modest elevation in the serum bilirubin and aminotransferases. A coagulopathy indicates that the liver insult is severe and the patient is at risk of acute liver failure. Most cases have an underlying procoagulant state that may be occult. The most frequent associations are:

• factor V Leiden
• *JAK3* gene mutation
• antiphospholipid antibody syndrome
• essential thrombocythemia
• polycythemia rubra vera
• antithrombin III deficiency
• protein C or S deficiency
• paroxysmal nocturnal hemoglobinuria.

Mechanical obstruction with cysts or tumors may precipitate the thrombosis; in Asians from the Far East, webs in the vena cava are a notable cause of Budd–Chiari syndrome.

The diagnosis is suggested by failure to demonstrate patent hepatic veins on ultrasonography or CT scanning and is confirmed by direct venography. A liver biopsy may be useful in identifying long-standing cases, and may reveal significant fibrosis or cirrhosis.

The usual treatment of acute Budd–Chiari syndrome is a decompressive shunt, fashioned either surgically or by construction of a transjugular intrahepatic portosystemic shunt (TIPS) (Figure 2.2). Liver transplantation is indicated in patients with established cirrhosis, those showing manifestations of acute liver failure and those whose condition deteriorates after shunting.

Veno-occlusive disease is clinically similar to the Budd–Chiari syndrome, but the main hepatic veins are patent and the obstruction occurs in the small hepatic venules. The disease may be caused by alkaloids (e.g. those present in bush tea and some chemotherapeutic agents); it also occurs after bone marrow transplantation. Management is similar to that of Budd–Chiari syndrome.

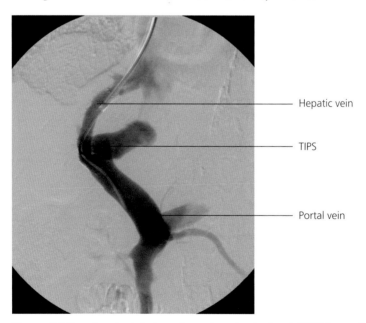

Hepatic vein

TIPS

Portal vein

Figure 2.2 Transjugular intrahepatic portosystemic shunt (TIPS) immediately after insertion, with catheter still in situ.

Key points – acute liver disease

- Attempt to classify acute liver disease as hepatitis (most common), cholestatic (intermediate) or vascular (unusual).
- Simple blood tests and an ultrasound examination provide most of the information required.
- Hypoglycemia, coagulopathy and any evidence of confusion indicate a high risk of acute liver failure and the need for specialist care.
- Coagulopathy in cholestatic disorders responds to parenteral vitamin K.

Key references

Lake JR, Sussman NL. Determining prognosis in patients with fulminant hepatic failure: when you absolutely, positively have to know the answer. *Hepatology* 1995;21:879–82.

Norris S. Drug- and toxin-induced liver damage. In: O'Grady JG, Lake JR, Howdle PD, eds. *Comprehensive Clinical Hepatology*. London: Mosby, 2000:ch 29.1, pp 1–20.

Valla D-C. The diagnosis and management of the Budd–Chiari syndrome: consensus and controversies. *Hepatology* 2003;38:793–803.

Alcoholic liver disease (ALD) is a common cause of end-stage liver disease, resulting in substantial morbidity and mortality throughout the world. In the USA, approximately 2 million people suffer from an alcohol-induced liver disorder. In the UK in 2012, ALD accounted for 63% (4425) of all alcohol-related deaths, an 18% increase on 2002. Medical costs associated with caring for these patients are enormous.

Alcohol-related liver injury presents a spectrum of disease, including asymptomatic hepatic steatosis (fatty liver), steatosis accompanied by inflammation (steatohepatitis or alcoholic hepatitis), cirrhosis with liver failure, variceal bleeding, ascites and even the development of hepatocellular carcinoma. Intervention for patients presenting with the early stages of liver injury helps to prevent further permanent liver injury. Interrupting alcoholism is the key, but this is not an easy task and frustrates many primary care providers, families and patients.

Diagnosis

Presentation. Patients may present anywhere along the spectrum of ALD. Those with isolated steatosis usually have few symptoms or signs of liver disease and are typically identified only by abnormal liver tests. Patients with alcoholic hepatitis are usually jaundiced and report fatigue, malaise and anorexia. The liver is enlarged and tender, and ascites and edema are often present. Patients with established cirrhosis usually display signs of portal hypertension, such as splenomegaly, caput medusae and ascites. In late-stage disease, the liver may be small and hard and there may be cutaneous stigmata of chronic liver disease, such as palmar erythema, spider nevi or telangiectasia (Figure 3.1). Gynecomastia and small shrunken testicles may be present in men. Diagnosis and treatment are summarized in Table 3.1.

Liver function tests. Examination of laboratory results is helpful in diagnosing ALD. The aminotransferases are elevated and have a

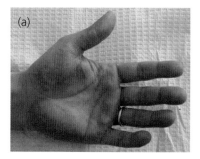
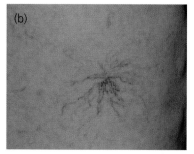

Figure 3.1 Cutaneous stigmata characteristic of alcohol-related liver damage: (a) palmar erythema, reproduced courtesy of the *Online Journal of Hepatology*; (b) spider nevus, reproduced courtesy of the Primary Care Dermatology Society.

characteristic pattern in patients with ALD: the aspartate aminotransferase (AST) is almost always higher than the alanine aminotransferase (ALT) level, and the greater the ratio the more likely that the liver disease is due to alcohol. Alkaline phosphatase and serum bilirubin levels may be increased, the prothrombin time (PT) prolonged and the albumin level depressed. The last two are good markers of the severity of ALD. However, it should also be noted that liver function tests may be entirely normal in the presence of cirrhosis, particularly if the patient has achieved sobriety.

Further investigations. Ultrasound or computed tomography (CT) images of the abdomen typically show parenchymal abnormalities suggestive of fatty changes in the liver (Figure 3.2), and may show a nodular outline typical of cirrhosis. Changes of portal hypertension, such as portosystemic collaterals and ascites, can also be seen on imaging studies. A liver biopsy is the gold standard for diagnosing ALD and in documenting the severity of liver injury, but may not be required in all cases. This is particularly true when the patient's history is suggestive of ALD, there is no evidence of viral hepatitis and biopsy could be difficult (i.e. patients with coagulopathy or severe ascites).

Concomitant disease. It is important to rule out other forms of liver disease and to document any concomitant injurious agents. Chronic

TABLE 3.1

Diagnosis and treatment of alcoholic liver disease

Alcoholic steatosis	Alcoholic hepatitis	Alcoholic cirrhosis
Symptoms		
Few, non-specific	Malaise, nausea, fatigue	Variable
Examination		
Hepatomegaly	Hepatomegaly, jaundice, ascites	Cutaneous stigmata of liver disease, portal hypertension
Laboratory tests		
AST > ALT, normal bilirubin, albumin and PT, GGT elevated	AST > ALT, WBCs elevated, bilirubin elevated, albumin depressed	PT elevated, bilirubin elevated, albumin depressed, platelet count low
Histology		
Steatosis	Steatosis with active inflammation	Fibrosis
Treatment		
Abstinence	Abstinence; aggressive nutrition, consider corticosteroids	Abstinence; treat complications

ALT, alanine aminotransferase; AST, aspartate aminotransferase; GGT, gamma-glutamyltransferase; PT, prothrombin time; WBC, white blood cell.

hepatitis C and, to a lesser extent, hepatitis B are common in patients with alcoholism. Although most patients who drink alcohol never develop significant liver disease, and many patients with viral hepatitis do well over long periods of time, the combination of viral hepatitis and alcoholism often accelerates the development of advanced liver injury. Thus, identification of a patient with both diseases is important.

There is an interesting parallel between ALD and the more recently recognized non-alcoholic fatty liver disease (NAFLD; see Chapter 6),

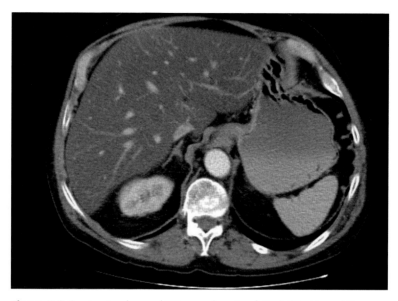

Figure 3.2 Contrast-enhanced CT scan showing fatty infiltration of the liver. Reproduced under a Creative Commons licence. CT scan by Prashanth Saddala, PERFUSE Study Group, Beth Israel Deaconess Medical Center, Harvard Medical School, USA. © 2012.

which is usually seen in patients with insulin resistance, obesity or diabetes. Both disorders are characterized by the deposition of fat (triglyceride) in the liver and progression through stages of inflammation to collagen deposition and fibrosis. Histologically, ALD and NAFLD appear identical, and some investigators feel that they differ only in the mechanism by which fat is originally deposited. Once fat appears in the liver, a similar progression of events occurs in some patients, resulting in irreversible scarring in the liver.

Determination of alcohol consumption. Although it seems self-evident, the diagnosis of ALD is made easier if it can be documented that the patient is drinking injurious amounts of alcohol (i.e. 80 g – about six drinks – per day for men and as little as 20 g per day for women). Accurate determination of alcohol consumption can be difficult, however, as patients often under-report how much alcohol they consume, and denial is common. The CAGE questionnaire, the

35

Alcohol Use Disorders Identification Test (AUDIT) and reports from families may be helpful in identifying patients whose alcohol consumption is excessive (see Table 1.2).

It should be remembered, however, that small amounts of alcohol (1–2 drinks per day) are probably beneficial, as has been reported extensively in the medical literature and popularized by the lay press.

Small amounts of alcohol would not be expected to cause ALD in men and, if it can be confirmed that a patient consumes only a small amount of alcohol, other causes of liver disease must be considered.

Treatment

The treatment of ALD essentially entails abstinence from alcohol, which is clearly the most important factor in promoting both short- and long-term survival. Achieving abstinence typically requires a multidisciplinary approach, involving organizations such as Alcoholics Anonymous, professional alcoholism counselors and, often, mental health professionals. This requires a substantial commitment on the part of the patient and the patient's family. Ideally, the patient will be encouraged by the knowledge that, with cessation of alcohol intake, their liver function is likely to improve substantially.

Nutrition. Alcoholics are usually malnourished, and improving nutrition is associated with improved outcomes. This is particularly important for patients with alcoholic hepatitis. Anorexia may prevent adequate nutrition and feeding via an enteral tube is sometimes required. Most alcoholics need protein. Unfortunately, however, a few patients with advanced liver disease develop hepatic encephalopathy when given large amounts of protein. Consultation with dietitians may be beneficial.

Corticosteroids. Alcoholic hepatitis is an inflammatory condition. Thus, corticosteroids are a logical treatment for ALD. However, despite many studies that have investigated the role of corticosteroids in the treatment of alcoholic hepatitis, there is no clear consensus on their efficacy. Most hepatologists believe that patients with the most severe forms of alcoholic hepatitis – i.e. those with a Maddrey's discriminant function (DF) score greater than 32 – will benefit from a course of corticosteroids. The DF score is calculated with the simple formula:

4.6 × [prothrombin time – control time (seconds)] + bilirubin (mg/dL)

To calculate the DF using bilirubin in SI units (micromol/L) divide the bilirubin value by 17.

Recent data suggest that short-term survival may be enhanced by infusions of N-acetylcysteine.

Tumor necrosis factor. Elevated levels of tumor necrosis factor (TNF) have been recorded in patients with alcoholic hepatitis, and clinical outcome appears to correlate with TNF levels. Efforts to decrease TNF levels have shown some promise in the treatment of patients with alcoholic hepatitis. One study has documented that pentoxifylline improved survival in patients with alcoholic hepatitis, presumably by interfering with TNF.

Liver transplantation for patients with ALD remains a controversial topic. Most transplant centers will consider patients with ALD as candidates for transplantation provided they have a documented period of abstinence from alcohol of at least 6 months before transplantation is considered. Unfortunately, some patients do return to drinking following transplant, although long-term success is common.

Key points – alcoholic liver disease

- Alcoholic liver disease (ALD) is a common cause of end-stage liver disease.
- Early intervention prevents permanent injury, but interrupting alcoholism can be difficult.
- Patients with ALD typically have mild to moderate elevations in aminotransferases, with AST > ALT.
- Patients with ALD are often malnourished; improving nutrition is an important treatment goal.
- Patients with severe alcoholic hepatitis may benefit from corticosteroids or pentoxifylline.

Key references

Babor TF, Biddle-Higgins JC, Saunders JB, Monteiro MG. AUDIT: *The Alcohol Use Disorders Identification Test: Guidelines for Use in Primary Health Care.* Geneva: World Health Organization, 2001. http://whqlibdoc.who.int/hq/2001/WHO_MSD_MSB_01.6a.pdf

Choi G, Runyon BA. Alcoholic hepatitis: a clinician's guide. *Clin Liver Dis* 2012;16:371.

European Association for the Study of the Liver. EASL clinical practical guidelines: management of alcoholic liver disease. *J Hepatol* 2012;57:3 99–420.

Ewing JA. Detecting alcoholism: the CAGE questionaire. *JAMA* 1984;252:1905–7.

Lucey MR, Mathurin P, Morgan TR. Alcoholic hepatitis. *N Engl J Med* 2009;360:2758–69.

Mathurin P, Moreno C, Samuel D et al. Early transplant for severe alcoholic hepatitis. *N Engl J Med* 2011;365:1790–800.

O'Shea RS, Dasarathy S, McCullough AJ. Alcoholic liver disease. *Am J Gastroenterol* 2010;105:14–32.

The liver is uniquely positioned, both anatomically and metabolically, to receive the brunt of potential insults; thus, medications have the potential to induce liver disease, and at least 1000 drugs have been implicated. Medications appear to be the cause of 50% of cases of acute liver failure in the USA, and as pharmacotherapy advances the treatment of many disorders, drug-induced liver injury (DILI) may also rise. The growing use of herbal preparations and traditional medicines is also of great concern. Whereas all approved medications have been evaluated at least superficially for hepatotoxicity, the majority of 'natural' remedies have not.

Prompt recognition of DILI is important because continued use of the drug often results in poor outcome. Unfortunately, other than the use of N-acetylcysteine for paracetamol (acetaminophen)-induced hepatotoxicity (see below), there are no specific 'antidotes' for DILI. Stopping the offending medication, supportive care and, in some circumstances, liver transplantation are the only treatments.

Diagnosis

DILI typically presents in one of three clinical patterns (Table 4.1). These presentations are similar or even identical to liver injuries from other causes. Thus, identification of DILI relies more on the history of exposure than on any particular finding on examination or from laboratory investigations. Specific medications typically produce a specific and reproducible pattern of liver injury, referred to as the hepatotoxicity profile of the drug.

Two general pathogenetic mechanisms are recognized.
- Predictable or direct DILI usually promptly follows an exposure to a new medication and appears to be due to direct toxicity or a toxic metabolite. Paracetamol is an example.
- Unpredictable or idiosyncratic DILI may be related to immune hypersensitivity: rash, fever and eosinophilia are typically present. These reactions follow a few weeks after exposure. Hepatotoxicity

TABLE 4.1

Clinical patterns of drug-induced liver disease

Cells injured	Presentation	Examples of causative drugs
Hepatitis-like		
Hepatocytes	Elevated aminotransferases	Paracetamol (acetaminophen), thiazolidinediones (e.g. pioglitazone, isoniazid), statins
Cholestasis		
Biliary canaliculi	Elevated alkaline phosphatase, pruritus	Chlorpromazine, erythromycin, estrogens
Mixed		
Biliary canaliculi and hepatocytes	Variable elevations in aminotransferases and alkaline phosphatase	Amoxicillin–clavulanic acid

due to amoxicillin–clavulanic acid is an example. Late-onset idiosyncratic reactions are difficult to recognize. They follow exposure by many months and usually do not display features of hypersensitivity. Isoniazid is an example.

Drugs commonly associated with hepatotoxicity

Statins (3-hydroxy-3-methylglutaryl coenzyme A [HMG-CoA] reductase inhibitors) reduce cardiovascular morbidity and mortality in patients with and without cardiovascular disease. These drugs are so effective that they are in very common use. As a group the statins are very safe, with fewer than 2% of patients enrolled in clinical trials discontinuing the medications for any reason. Nevertheless, elevation of the aminotransferases (greater than three times normal) occurs in approximately 1% of exposed patients. Lesser elevations in the aminotransferases are more common (i.e. about 3%). The effect appears to be dose-related and usually occurs in the first few months of therapy. Most patients are asymptomatic and have no signs suggestive of liver dysfunction on physical examination. Severe liver injury has been reported but is rare.

Periodic monitoring of liver tests is recommended, although there is no evidence that monitoring prevents serious liver disease. The abnormalities are generally not progressive and may resolve despite continued use of the drug. Nevertheless, if significant persistent elevations in liver tests occur, the statin should be discontinued. Starting a different statin once the liver abnormalities have resolved, and monitoring the patient's liver tests for a period, is appropriate.

A common clinical question is whether to use a statin in a patient with pre-existing liver disease. Unfortunately, there is little evidence on which to make an informed decision. A retrospective study found that patients with baseline elevated aminotransferases were no more likely to develop further elevation in liver tests when taking a statin than were patients with abnormal aminotransferases who were not taking statins. Thus, it is probably acceptable to use the statins in patients with chronic stable liver disease, provided symptoms and liver tests are monitored. Statins are contraindicated in patients with acute liver disease and those with advanced chronic liver disease (elevated bilirubin, depressed albumin, clinically apparent cirrhosis, etc.).

Paracetamol (acetaminophen) is a remarkably safe drug, but in certain circumstances it has significant hepatotoxicity.

- Doses greater than approximately 10 g, usually taken as a suicide attempt, are a well-known cause of liver failure.
- Lower doses, typically used without suicidal intent, can induce severe liver injury in patients who chronically use alcohol or who are malnourished. In these patients, doses within the therapeutic range (i.e. about 4 g) may be hepatotoxic.

Although non-specific symptoms such as nausea, vomiting and malaise are common within a few hours, patients typically have little evidence of liver injury until 24–48 hours after ingesting injurious amounts of paracetamol. The aminotransferases rise, occasionally peaking above

10 000 IU/L, and bilirubin is usually modestly elevated. Prothrombin time (PT), however, is often markedly prolonged. Right upper quadrant abdominal pain and signs of hepatic encephalopathy may develop. Renal failure is often seen. The clinical and laboratory abnormalities usually reach their peak by 3–4 days. For those who survive, recovery is usually prompt and complete and with no long-term sequelae to acute paracetamol liver injury.

The potential for hepatotoxicity following ingestion can be calculated using the Rumack–Matthew paracetamol nomogram (Figure 4.1). Serum paracetamol levels (drawn at least 4 hours after ingestion) are plotted against the time since ingestion. Patients with intersects below the line in the nomogram are at little risk for hepatotoxicity. It should be noted that the Rumack–Matthew nomogram may be inaccurate if overdose is with one of the many extended-release preparations now available.

Treatment. Activated charcoal should be given when the patient presents within 8 hours of ingestion. N-acetylcysteine is the definitive treatment for paracetamol overdose. It serves as a glutathione

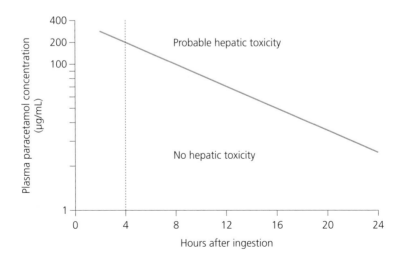

Figure 4.1 The Rumack–Matthew nomogram is used to calculate the potential for hepatotoxicity following ingestion of standard paracetamol (acetaminophen) tablets.

precursor, promoting the elimination of N-acetylbenzoquinoneimine, a hepatotoxic metabolite of paracetamol. Significant hepatotoxicity is uncommon when N-acetylcysteine is given within 8 hours of overdose. It is therefore imperative that N-acetylcysteine is given early (typically while awaiting paracetamol serum levels) and continued if significant hepatotoxicity has developed. If the nomogram suggests little chance of hepatotoxicity, N-acetylcysteine can be discontinued.

Although N-acetylcysteine can be administered orally, it is not palatable and has been replaced by an intravenous preparation that is now widely available. An infusion of 150 mg/kg (loading dose) is given over 15 minutes, followed by 50 mg/kg infusion over 4 hours, and the last 100 mg/kg is infused over the remaining 16 hours.

The development of progressive liver failure with encephalopathy mandates the transfer of the patient to a liver transplant center.

Isoniazid is a mainstay of treatment for both active and latent tuberculosis. Two types of hepatotoxicity are recognized. The first, and by far most common, is a transient mild elevation in the aminotransferases within a few months of beginning therapy. This occurs in approximately 20% of patients, who remain asymptomatic. Isoniazid should be continued and the patient monitored for symptoms and worsening liver tests. Often the liver test abnormalities will resolve despite continuing isoniazid.

Clinically evident isoniazid hepatitis, the second and much more serious form, is rare, occurring in less than 1% of treated patients. Fatal reactions are very rare (about 0.023%). About half of patients with clinical isoniazid hepatitis will develop symptoms within a few months of starting the drug, although presentations after as long as 12 months have been reported. The presentation is similar to acute viral hepatitis, so these infections should be excluded. Isoniazid should be stopped immediately and the patient observed closely. Ideally, an alternative tuberculosis regimen should be substituted after the hepatitis resolves.

At a minimum, patients who start taking isoniazid should be educated to recognize and report any symptoms suggestive of liver dysfunction. Patients with symptoms should be evaluated promptly and thoroughly. Guidelines for monitoring asymptomatic patients for hepatotoxicity vary. The US Centers for Disease Control recommend liver tests before treatment and then periodically during treatment only in patients at high risk for hepatotoxicity (Table 4.2). Others, reasoning that concomitant use of other drugs with hepatotoxic potential (rifampicin [rifampin] and pyrazinamide) is so common, recommend liver tests at regular intervals.

TABLE 4.2

Risk factors for severe isoniazid hepatotoxicity

- Patient < 5 years or > 35 years of age
- Alcoholism
- Pre-existing liver disease (viral hepatitis)
- Acquired immunodeficiency syndrome (AIDS)
- Concomitant use of rifampicin (rifampin) and/or pyrazinamide (both of which have been reported to cause liver injury)

Key points – drug-induced liver injury

- Drug-induced liver injury is common and usually mild.
- Determining the temporal relationship between starting a drug and the development of symptoms and signs of liver disease is important.
- Discontinuation of offending agents usually results in prompt resolution of hepatic injury.
- Monitoring for hepatotoxicity may be appropriate for some medications, such as statins and isoniazid.

Key references

Abboud G, Kaplowitz N. Drug-induced liver injury. *Drug Saf* 2007;30:277–94.

Bernal W, Wendon J. Acute liver failure. *N Engl J Med* 2013;369:2525–34.

O'Grady JG, Alexander GJ, Hayllar KM, Williams R. Early indicators of prognosis in fulminant hepatic failure. *Gastroenterology* 1989;97:439–45.

Stine JG, Lewis JH. Hepatotoxicity of antibiotics: a review and update for the clinician. *Clin Liver Dis* 2013;17:609–42.

Stravitz RT, Kramer DJ. Management of acute liver failure. *Nat Rev Gastroenterol Hepatol* 2009;6:542–53.

Tajiri K, Shimizu Y. Practical guidelines for diagnosis and early management of drug-induced liver injury. *World J Gastroenterol* 2008;14:6774–85.

Three liver diseases are categorized as autoimmune in etiology:

- autoimmune hepatitis (AIH), which targets the hepatocyte
- primary biliary cirrhosis (PBC), which affects the microscopic bile ducts
- primary sclerosing cholangitis (PSC), which can involve any elements of the intrahepatic and extrahepatic biliary system.

AIH and PBC are predominantly autoimmune diseases, but the categorization is less clear-cut with PSC. The classic immunologic profiles associated with these conditions are shown in Table 5.1. Some diagnostic confusion can occur because of the existence of 'overlap syndromes' or histological progression from apparent AIH to either PBC or PSC.

Autoimmune hepatitis

AIH is a chronic inflammatory liver disease of at least 6 months' duration. The target cell for the immunologic response is the

TABLE 5.1

Immunologic profiles in autoimmune liver diseases

Antibody	AIH	PBC	PSC
Antinuclear	++	+	++
Anti-smooth-muscle	+++	–	–
Anti-LKM*	+++	–	–
Antimitochondrial	–	+++	–
Elevated IgG	+++	–	+
Elevated IgM	–	++	–

–, not found; +, ++ and +++ indicate relative levels of antibodies.
*Type 2 AIH.
AIH, autoimmune hepatitis; Ig, immunoglobulin; LKM, liver–kidney microsomal; PBC, primary biliary cirrhosis; PSC, primary sclerosing cholangitis.

hepatocyte, and the dominant effector cells are lymphocytes and plasma cells. Two types of AIH are defined by classic autoantibody profiles:

- type 1: anti-smooth-muscle antibodies with or without antinuclear factor
- type 2: anti-liver-kidney microsomal antibodies.

These antibodies are associated with hypergammaglobulinemia, with a dominant elevation in the immunoglobulin (Ig) G fraction in untreated disease. Histological verification and staging of the disease is mandatory. The classic finding on liver histology is portal inflammation, with plasma cells and lymphocytes spilling over into the lobule in a pattern called interface hepatitis (Figure 5.1). Fibrosis or cirrhosis may be established by the time of presentation or may develop during follow-up despite apparently adequate therapy.

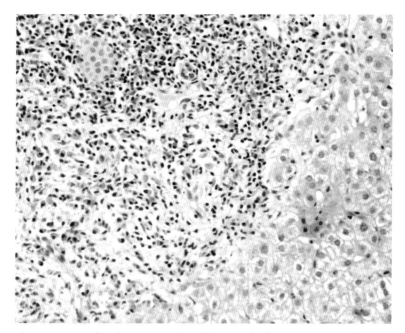

Figure 5.1 Interface hepatitis with 'spill-over' of inflammatory cells from the portal tract through the limiting plate into the liver parenchyma. This is the histological hallmark of untreated chronic autoimmune hepatitis. (Magnification × 200; picture courtesy of Dr A Knisley.)

Clinical features. There is a strong gender association, with 70% of cases occurring in women. The age at presentation has a bimodal distribution, with peaks during the second decade and the fourth and fifth decades.

AIH can present as an acute hepatitis-like illness, with jaundice and a laboratory profile showing hyperbilirubinemia and a marked elevation in serum aminotransferases (transaminases). A liver biopsy will show the characteristic features, with or without fibrosis or cirrhosis. Alternatively, patients may present with established cirrhosis in the absence of any previous episode of jaundice or other symptoms alerting to the presence of chronic hepatitis. These patients may present with liver failure or complications of portal hypertension. As with all causes of cirrhosis, there is a risk of hepatocellular carcinoma, but this risk is at the lower end of the spectrum in this condition.

Treatment. The standard treatment for AIH is immunosuppression with corticosteroids and azathioprine. Initial control is achieved with corticosteroids (e.g. prednisone, 30–60 mg/day). The dose is gradually reduced over 2–3 months to a target dose of 5–10 mg/day. Azathioprine is added as a steroid-sparing strategy and can be effective in maintaining remission, even after complete withdrawal of corticosteroids. Newer immunosuppressive drugs, such as mycophenolate and tacrolimus, are being used in refractory cases, but are not considered standard treatments for AIH.

The serum aminotransferases and IgG levels are used to monitor response to therapy. However, the intensity of necro-inflammatory activity may be understated by the serum aminotransferase levels, and repeat biopsy is recommended to confirm disease remission or if withdrawal of immunosuppressive therapy is being considered. Flares in disease activity occur in patients on stable long-term therapy and after reductions in drug dose. These flares are treated in a similar way to newly diagnosed disease.

Liver transplantation is an effective therapy for advanced disease. AIH recurs in up to 40% of cases but is generally easily controlled by inclusion of a higher dose of corticosteroids in the maintenance immunosuppression regimen.

Primary biliary cirrhosis

PBC is a progressive disease with an asymptomatic phase that may last for 15–20 years. The asymptomatic phase is being increasingly recognized, however, with the detection of increased alkaline phosphatase levels on routine blood tests. The diagnosis is effectively established by the detection of positive antimitochondrial antibodies (AMA), usually of the M2 subtype. The IgM fraction of the serum gammaglobulins is normally raised. The combination of elevated alkaline phosphatase, positive AMA and elevated IgM is now considered diagnostic of PBC; histological verification is no longer necessary. However, a liver biopsy may be of value in staging the severity of the disease.

Clinical features. The first symptoms are usually pruritus (itch) and lethargy (tiredness). The cause of the itch is unclear, but it responds in many cases to therapies that deplete bile salts (e.g. colestyramine [cholestyramine]). Antihistamines are not effective in this situation. The therapies used to treat the pruritus are listed in Table 5.2. The cause of the lethargy is also unclear, but there is increasing evidence to suggest that it is 'central' and secondary to changes within the brain. Hypothyroidism develops in up to 20% of patients with PBC, so it is important to screen regularly for this as a cause of the lethargy.

The development of jaundice indicates that the disease is entering the final stage, which lasts for 3–5 years.

The prolonged cholestasis leads to cholesterol deposition in the skin (xanthomas and xanthelasma) and osteopenia or osteoporosis

TABLE 5.2

Treatments used for pruritus in primary biliary cirrhosis

- Colestyramine (cholestyramine)
- Ursodeoxycholic acid
- Rifampicin (rifampin)
- Naltrexone
- Ondansetron

(Figure 5.2). At this stage, patients may also exhibit signs of portal hypertension, with ascites and esophageal or gastric varices. Encephalopathy is less common than in other causes of end-stage chronic liver disease.

Treatment. There is no curative medical therapy for PBC. There is some evidence to support treatment with ursodeoxycholic acid (UDCA), as this improves the biochemical profile and possibly the histological appearance. There is, however, limited evidence that UDCA prolongs survival or delays the need for liver transplantation.

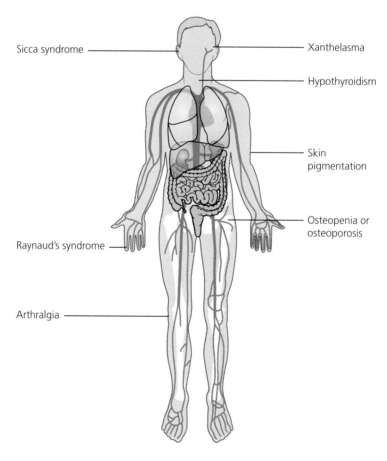

Sicca syndrome

Xanthelasma

Hypothyroidism

Skin pigmentation

Osteopenia or osteoporosis

Raynaud's syndrome

Arthralgia

Figure 5.2 Extrahepatic associations in primary biliary cirrhosis.

A number of other immunosuppressive and antifibrotic therapies have failed to demonstrate sufficient benefit to gain widespread use.

Liver transplantation is still the only effective treatment for advanced PBC. The indications for transplantation are liver failure, defined by the Model for End-Stage Liver Disease (MELD) as a disease severity score ranging from 4 to 40, typically above 20; severe and intractable pruritus; and hepatocellular carcinoma The results of liver transplantation for PBC are excellent. There is evidence that PBC recurs in the transplanted liver, but this phenomenon appears to be of little clinical relevance in the first 10–15 years after transplantation.

Primary sclerosing cholangitis

PSC can affect all elements of the biliary system.

Diagnosis. Cholangiography classically shows diffuse stricturing and beading involving both the intrahepatic and extrahepatic bile ducts. In some cases, the extrahepatic bile ducts are spared, which reduces the confidence in making the diagnosis on radiological criteria.

Liver histology may show the characteristic lesion of concentric fibrosis around the small bile ducts, termed 'onion-skin' fibrosis. The characteristic autoantibody is perinuclear antineutrophil cytoplasmic antibody (pANCA), but other autoantibodies may also be detected.

Clinical features. There is a strong association between PSC and inflammatory disease involving the large bowel – mainly ulcerative colitis but also Crohn's disease. About 75% of patients with PSC have inflammatory bowel disease and up to 7.5% of patients with ulcerative colitis have PSC. The diagnosis of PSC may be suggested by the detection of elevated cholestatic enzymes, particularly alkaline phosphatase, on routine screening of patients with inflammatory bowel disease. More advanced disease presents with jaundice and symptoms of biliary obstruction (dark urine, pale stools, itch) or low-grade cholangitis (fevers, sweats, feeling intermittently hot and cold).

Natural history. This is less predictable than that of PBC. Fluctuations in disease may:
- settle spontaneously
- respond to antibiotic therapy
- respond to treatment with UDCA
- improve after endoscopic dilation of a dominant stricture.

A rapid deterioration may indicate the development of a complicating cholangiocarcinoma. The risk of this malignant transformation is about 6–15% over the course of the disease. Screening for malignant transformation is not effective in detecting early disease, and progression to cholangiocarcinoma is generally regarded as a contraindication to liver transplantation.

Treatment. UDCA, 10–15 mg/kg/day, is recommended. This ameliorates pruritus, improves the liver biochemistry and histology and may alter the natural history of the disease. Immunosuppressive and antifibrotic therapies have not proved effective.

Liver transplantation is used widely for advanced disease. The indications for transplantation are less precise than they are in PBC, but persistent jaundice of more than 3 months' duration, in addition to evidence of liver failure or severe portal hypertension, are reasonable indications to proceed to liver transplantation. The results of liver transplantation are excellent in the absence of cholangiocarcinoma. PSC recurs in 8–15% of cases and is occasionally a cause of significant graft dysfunction.

Overlap syndromes

Diagnostic confusion may arise in some patients who manifest features of more than one autoimmune disease. Patients with early PBC may have florid interface hepatitis on liver biopsy, but this should not be confused with AIH. Other patients have features of AIH and a cholangiopathy, and these are considered to have an 'overlap syndrome' or autoimmune cholangiopathy. These patients are managed as if they had both diseases (i.e. with corticosteroids and UDCA).

Key points – autoimmune liver diseases

- Autoimmune liver disease can target the hepatocyte or any element of the bile duct system.
- Autoimmune hepatitis (AIH) is potentially treatable if diagnosed before the development of cirrhosis.
- Primary biliary cirrhosis (PBC) is a slowly progressive disease, with a presymptomatic period of up to 20 years.
- Liver transplantation is an excellent treatment for end-stage AIH and PBC.
- Primary sclerosing cholangitis is strongly associated with ulcerative colitis and is unpredictable; late disease can be managed effectively with liver transplantation unless complicated by cholangiocarcinoma.

Key references

Durazzo M, Premoli A, Fagoonee S, Pellicano R. Overlap syndromes of autoimmune hepatitis: what is known so far. *Dig Dis Sci* 2003;48: 423–30.

Levy C, Lindor KD. Current management of primary biliary cirrhosis and primary sclerosing cholangitis. *J Hepatol* 2003;38: S24–37.

McFarlane IG. Autoimmune hepatitis: diagnostic criteria, subclassifications, and clinical features. *Clin Liver Dis* 2002;6: 317–33.

Poupon RE, Lindor KD, Cauch-Dudek K et al. Combined analysis of randomised controlled trials of ursodeoxycholic acid in primary biliary cirrhosis. *Gastroenterology* 1997;113:884–90.

Talwalkar JA, Lindor KD. Primary biliary cirrhosis. *Lancet* 2003:362;53–61.

Non-alcoholic fatty liver disease

Non-alcoholic fatty liver disease (NAFLD) is a group of disorders of diverse etiology (Table 6.1) and presents as a spectrum of disease ranging from apparently innocuous deposition of fat in the liver to cirrhosis with liver failure. Once thought to be uncommon and benign, NAFLD is now recognized as one of the most common forms of serious liver disease in Western populations. The growing prevalence of disorders associated with NAFLD (particularly diabetes, obesity and hyperlipidemia) suggests that fatty liver disease will be an important cause of morbidity and even mortality in the future. This discussion focuses on steatosis associated with insulin resistance.

Simple steatosis is the initial, and presumably most benign, type of NAFLD. Microscopically, fat droplets are seen in the hepatocytes and there is no or minimal inflammatory component. Simple steatosis is the most predictable form of fatty liver disease, occurring in many patients with diabetes and/or obesity. In the second, more advanced stage, an inflammatory response accompanies the fat. This lesion is termed non-alcoholic steatohepatitis (NASH). The liver cells swell and are surrounded by inflammatory cells. The most advanced stages of NAFLD are marked by deposition of collagen in the liver, resulting in progressive fibrosis and eventually the architectural distortion that

TABLE 6.1

Common conditions associated with fatty liver

- Insulin resistance
  - diabetes
  - obesity
  - hyperlipidemia
- Starvation and rapid weight loss
- Parenteral nutrition
- Medications
  - corticosteroids
  - methotrexate
  - amiodarone
  - antiretrovirals

signifies cirrhosis. These later two stages are unpredictable and develop from simple steatosis in a minority of patients.

Pathogenesis. The pathogenesis of NAFLD is incompletely understood. Insulin resistance plays an important role in the disease of the majority of patients with hepatic steatosis, namely those with obesity, hypertension, diabetes and hyperlipidemia. Insulin resistance results in a complex cascade of events that increases triglyceride delivery to, and decreases triglyceride secretion from, the liver. The net result is accumulation of fat in the hepatocytes. How simple steatosis develops into inflammation and fibrosis is not known. One theory suggests that mitochondrial fatty acid metabolism leads to the production of reactive oxygen species, which results in lipid peroxidation. Altered lipids are substrates for immune attack, which promotes the elaboration of cytokines from immune effector cells, leading to further cell injury. Peroxidized lipids and cytokines appear to promote activation of collagen-producing stellate cells, eventually resulting in cirrhosis.

Clinical presentation and diagnosis. Most patients with the early stages of NAFLD have few symptoms and are typically first identified by abnormal liver tests on routine screening. Hepatomegaly may be noted, but unless cirrhosis has developed with portal hypertension and/or liver failure, the examination is often unrevealing. The aminotransferases are usually mildly elevated, with alanine aminotransferase (ALT) typically higher than aspartate aminotransferase (AST) – an important characteristic.

As there is no specific laboratory test for NAFLD, most practitioners make a tentative diagnosis by excluding other causes of liver disease. Negative serology for hepatitis B and C rule out these chronic viral infections. Negative antinuclear and anti-smooth-muscle antibodies help rule out autoimmune hepatitis (AIH, see Chapter 5). Inquiry regarding the use of prescribed and over-the-counter medications and nutritional supplements, particularly if there is a known temporal association between drug use and liver injury, helps to eliminate drug-induced injury (DILI, see Chapter 4). The possibility of drug-induced liver disease warrants attention, given that many patients take a variety of medications for disorders associated with NAFLD (diabetes, obesity and hyperlipidemia), and some of these medications have been reported to cause hepatic injury.

Without a definitive method to quantify alcohol intake accurately, separating alcoholic liver disease (ALD) from NAFLD remains problematic; histologically, they may be indistinguishable. The aminotransferase ratio – ALT higher than AST – and an accurate history from the patient and family members are helpful. However, the cautious physician will remember that obtaining an accurate alcohol history is quite difficult.

Imaging studies (ultrasonography and computed tomography) can detect significant hepatic steatosis. However, these studies cannot determine if inflammation or fibrosis accompanies the fat. There is currently no consensus on which patients require a liver biopsy to confirm the diagnosis of NAFLD. Many healthcare providers feel that in the appropriate patient (i.e. with obesity, diabetes and hyperlipidemia), in whom other disorders have been eliminated, the diagnosis of NAFLD is likely and a biopsy would be unlikely to alter treatment. It should be recognized, however, that the advanced forms of NAFLD cannot be reliably separated from simple fat without a biopsy. Thus, liver biopsy still plays an important role both in the ultimate diagnosis of the disorder and in determining prognosis.

Natural history. The natural history of NAFLD is incompletely defined. Early descriptions of the disorder suggested that the course was essentially benign, whereas current evidence is less optimistic. Many patients have an uneventful course; however, some will advance to end-stage liver disease and are vulnerable to all the complications of cirrhosis. Unfortunately, the comorbid conditions provoked by insulin resistance (atherosclerosis, kidney disease) make these patients relatively poor candidates for liver transplantation should they develop advancing liver failure.

Treatment. Weight reduction is the mainstay of treatment for NAFLD. Patients should be strongly encouraged to lose weight slowly, as there is some evidence to suggest that rapid weight loss may provoke inflammation and even liver failure. Unfortunately, weight loss is extraordinarily difficult for most patients and success is often not achieved. However, the patient should be encouraged with the knowledge that weight loss is almost always associated with an improvement in liver tests and perhaps liver function (see *Fast Facts: Obesity*). Careful control of diabetes and hyperlipidemia is recommended, although this may not affect the underlying liver disease (see *Fast Facts: Diabetes Mellitus* and *Fast Facts: Hyperlipidemia*).

Currently, no medications are universally accepted to alter the course of NAFLD. The insulin-sensitizing medications are logical choices. Promising results have been seen with vitamin E (1000 units daily) and pioglitazone, and these agents should be considered if weight loss fails. Bariatric surgery appears to be effective.

Hemochromatosis

Hemochromatosis is an inherited disorder of iron overload. Although common, it is underdiagnosed. It is now possible to test for the genetic markers associated with this disorder, and we hope that these tests will alter diagnostic acumen and lead to early discovery and treatment of patients with the condition.

Pathogenesis. The proximal intestine regulates iron balance.
• When there is a relative systemic deficiency of iron, absorption of iron from food is facilitated.
• When body stores are replete, absorption is downregulated and iron balance is maintained.
• There is no normal process for eliminating excessive body iron. Genetic mutations associated with hemochromatosis result in altered regulation of iron absorption. The mutated gene product interferes with the cellular reporting of normal iron levels leading to the perception of iron deficiency, and the downregulation of iron absorption that normally accompanies the iron-replete state does not occur. Rather, iron absorption continues and iron is deposited in a variety of body tissues. A newly described protein hepcidin plays an important role.

In hemochromatosis, unregulated iron absorption continues uninterrupted from birth. Critical tissue levels of iron (levels high enough to initiate injury) are reached after more than 30 years, first in

57

men and later in women (who are somewhat 'protected' while they lose iron during menstruation).

Excess iron appears to promote the generation of oxygen free radicals, which interact with lipid-rich membranes to form lipid peroxides. This results in membrane damage, cell death and promotion of fibrosis. After years of uncontrolled iron accumulation and injury, extensive fibrosis (cirrhosis) develops, resulting in organ dysfunction.

Clinical presentation. Most patients with hemochromatosis complain of fatigue and some will report arthralgia and loss of libido. Unfortunately, however, hemochromatosis has no specific symptoms and the disease is usually not suspected until significant, often irreversible, organ damage has occurred. Excessive iron is deposited in many organs and causes injury (Table 6.2). Age (older), gender (men), alcohol abuse, oral iron intake (supplements) and infection with hepatitis C may potentiate disease expression.

Diagnosis. The key to diagnosing hemochromatosis is to have a high index of suspicion. Unexplained cirrhosis or heart failure (particularly

TABLE 6.2

Manifestations of hemochromatosis

Organ	Result
Liver	Cirrhosis Hepatocellular carcinoma
Heart	Pump failure* Arrhythmia*
Pancreas	Diabetes*
Skin	Increased pigmentation*
Pituitary	Hypogonadism
Joints	Arthritis – metacarpophalangeal joints

*Possibly reversible with treatment.

if diabetes is present) should raise concern. Often, abnormal iron levels are the only indication of the disease. Liver function tests (AST, ALT and alkaline phosphatase) are typically normal or only slightly elevated. Liver functional parameters are non-specific and reflect the severity of liver dysfunction. Blood glucose levels may be elevated, reflecting destruction of pancreatic islets.

Transferrin saturation is a better diagnostic tool than ferritin concentration, which is often elevated in inflammatory conditions and non-hemochromatosis liver disorders. A transferrin saturation (serum iron divided by transferrin concentration) greater than 50% is suggestive of hemochromatosis. A ferritin concentration greater than twice the upper limit of normal deserves further investigation (Table 6.3). Studies have shown that elevated iron levels are not uncommon in the population; persistent values are the most suggestive of true iron overload.

Genetic tests. The *HFE* (High Fe) gene plays an important role in the regulation of iron absorption. Mutations in this gene are associated with hemochromatosis, and blood tests for the gene are commercially available. The most common mutation is cysteine to tyrosine at residue 282 (C282Y mutation) and is seen in most patients with the disease. Single copies of the mutation are relatively common in unselected populations (approximately 2%) but are much more

TABLE 6.3

Tests for hemochromatosis

Laboratory test	Hemochromatosis	Normal
Transferrin saturation (%)	> 50%	15–45
Ferritin (ng/dL)	> 600	< 300
Genetic markers	C282Y/C282Y	
Hepatic iron (mmol/g liver)	> 70	< 40
Hepatic iron index*	> 1.9	< 1.5

* The hepatic iron index is calculated by dividing the hepatic iron concentration by the patient's age.

common in some ethnic groups (approximately 10% of Irish). A histidine-to-aspartic-acid mutation at residue 63 (the H63D mutation) has also been described and appears to be more common but less severe than the C282Y mutation.

Patients who are homozygous for the C282Y mutation (C282Y/C282Y) are at greatest risk for significant iron overload and end-organ damage, whereas patients with one copy of each mutation (C282Y/H63D) are at less risk. Patients who are heterozygous for the C282Y mutation typically do not develop pathological iron overload. The clinical significance of homozygosity for the H63D mutation (H63D/H63D) has been questioned – it may not predispose to pathological iron overload.

It is important to recognize that not all patients with hemochromatosis have typical mutations. Similarly, not all patients with typical mutations will develop pathological iron overload – the penetration of the mutations is not yet fully understood.

Liver biopsy can be helpful in diagnosing hemochromatosis, as iron can be directly determined in a biopsy sample by chemical methods. A hepatic iron index, calculated by dividing the hepatic iron concentration by the patient's age, is regarded as the gold standard for the diagnosis of the disorder. Iron stains show excessive parenchymal deposition of iron, but this method is, at best, semiquantitative. The hepatology community is divided on the need to perform a liver biopsy to confirm the diagnosis in patients suspected of having hemochromatosis on the basis of serum iron studies and/or genetic tests. In general, it is recommended that patients with abnormal liver blood tests or other signs of liver disease undergo liver biopsy to confirm the diagnosis and determine the presence and severity of fibrosis.

Treatment. Reduction of systemic iron overload is the foundation of management for hemochromatosis. Therapeutic phlebotomy (Table 6.4), involving removal of one unit of blood (approximately 500 mL) approximately once a week, is necessary until the patient is iron-deficient (ferritin < 50 ng/dL). Once iron deficiency is achieved, the frequency of phlebotomy can be reduced to once every 2–4 months to maintain a low ferritin concentration. Alcohol consumption and

TABLE 6.4

Phlebotomy protocol for the management of hemochromatosis

- Stop all iron supplements and limit alcohol intake
- Begin phlebotomy:
  - remove one unit of blood (approximately 500 mL) every week*
  - check hematocrit before each phlebotomy; proceed if > 35%
  - continue until ferritin < 50 ng/dL (usually 1 year!)
- Once ferritin < 50 ng/dL, reduce phlebotomies to every 2–4 months
- Adjust phlebotomy schedule to keep ferritin < 50 ng/dL; continue for life

*Some blood banks accept blood from patients with hemochromatosis.

iron supplements should be avoided, as should vitamin C supplements, as vitamin C facilitates iron absorption. Some physicians recommend oral antioxidants (vitamin E in particular) to help ameliorate iron-induced oxidation.

Hepatocellular carcinoma. Patients with hemochromatosis, particularly men with fibrotic disease, are at significant risk for hepatocellular carcinoma. It is reasonable to screen all patients with cirrhosis periodically (e.g. every 6 months) with serum alpha fetoprotein determination and ultrasound imaging of the liver.

Screening for hemochromatosis. Because hemochromatosis is an easily treatable autosomal dominant disorder but has potentially devastating consequences, screening for the disorder is appealing. Early diagnosis allows for reduction of iron overload before injury occurs. Close relatives of patients identified with hemochromatosis should be screened by measuring transferrin saturation and genetic markers.

There is currently no consensus on screening the general population for hemochromatosis, although it appears logical to screen populations with the highest prevalence of the disease (those of northern European decent). A single measurement of transferrin saturation at 30 years of age in men and 40 years of age in women may be appropriate in these groups.

Wilson's disease

Wilson's disease is an autosomal recessive disorder of copper homeostasis. The defect involves mutation in the gene that codes for a canalicular copper 'pump', leading to impaired excretion of copper into bile. Excessive accumulation of copper in the liver, brain and other tissues leads to organ dysfunction (Table 6.5). The disorder is uncommon (1 in 30 000) and affects all races.

Clinical presentation. Symptoms and signs of Wilson's disease typically develop in older children and young adults, although in a few patients the disease is not discovered until the fifth or sixth decade. Younger patients usually present with hepatic dysfunction, whereas neuropsychiatric manifestations dominate the presentation of older patients.

TABLE 6.5

Clinical manifestations of copper deposition in Wilson's disease

Organ	Clinical manifestations of copper deposition
Liver	Asymptomatic elevation of liver function tests
	Acute/chronic hepatitis
	Fulminant hepatic failure
	Cirrhosis
Brain	Tremor
	Ataxia
	Personality change/depression
Eye	Kayser–Fleischer rings
Red blood cells	Hemolysis
Kidney	Proximal renal tubular acidosis
	Hypouricemia

TABLE 6.6

Diagnostic tests for Wilson's disease

Test	Wilson's disease	Normal
Ceruloplasmin concentration	< 20 mg/dL	20–45 mg/dL
24-hour urinary copper excretion	> 100 µg	< 35 µg
Hepatic copper concentration	> 250 µg/g liver	< 50 µg/g liver

Diagnosis of Wilson's disease rests on maintaining a high degree of suspicion for the disorder. All young patients with abnormal liver tests, signs of liver disease or any unexplained neuropsychiatric disorder deserve investigation. Serum ceruloplasmin is low in 95% of patients with Wilson's disease. Definitive diagnosis rests on documenting excessive hepatic copper by liver biopsy (Table 6.6).

Treatment. The mainstay of treatment involves chelation of copper, allowing for urinary excretion. Penicillamine is the drug of choice, and trientine is used for the 30% of patients who are intolerant of penicillamine. Oral zinc appears to interfere with copper absorption by the small bowel and has been used as an adjunct to chelation therapy.

α_1 antitrypsin deficiency

α_1 antitrypsin deficiency (ATD) is a well-known cause of chronic lung disease. It is also associated with liver disease in children and adults. Although ATD is not rare (it affects approximately 1 in 1800 births), only a small percentage of patients with ATD will develop liver disease.

Diagnosis. The hepatic manifestations of ATD are listed in Table 6.7. Low serum levels of α_1 antitrypsin, a consistent protease inhibitor phenotype (i.e. protease inhibitor homozygous for the Z mutation;

63

PiZZ) and a liver biopsy that reveals granules in hepatocytes on periodic acid–Schiff (PAS) staining confirm the diagnosis.

Treatment. There is no specific treatment for ATD liver disease. Transplant is an option for patients with advanced liver disease provided their lungs have not been too severely affected.

TABLE 6.7

Hepatic manifestations of α_1 antitrypsin deficiency

Children	Adults
• Coagulopathy	• Chronic hepatitis
• Protracted jaundice	• Cirrhosis
• Neonatal hepatitis	• Hepatocellular carcinoma

Key points – metabolic liver diseases

- Non-alcoholic fatty liver disease (NAFLD) is a common liver disorder, most often seen in obese or diabetic patients.
- NAFLD is a spectrum of conditions from simple steatosis to cirrhosis with liver failure.
- When associated with obesity, NAFLD is best treated with weight loss.
- Hemochromatosis is easily treatable but underdiagnosed.
- It is reasonable to screen patients at risk of hemochromatosis by measuring the transferrin saturation in early middle age.

Key references

Allen KJ, Gurrin LC, Constantine CC et al. Iron-overload-related disease in HFE hereditary hemochromatosis. *N Engl J Med* 2008;358:221–30.

Bacon BR, Adams PC, Kowdley KV et al. Diagnosis and management of hemochromatosis: 2011 practice guideline by the American Association for the Study of Liver Diseases. *Hepatology* 2011;54: 328–43.

Chalasani N, Younossi Z, Lavine JE et al. The diagnosis and management of non-alcoholic fatty liver disease: practice Guideline by the American Association for the Study of Liver Diseases, American College of Gastroenterology, and the American Gastroenterological Association. *Hepatology* 2012;55:2005–23.

European Association for the Study of the Liver. EASL clinical practice guidelines for HFE hemochromatosis. *J Hepatol* 2010;53:3–22.

European Association for Study of Liver. EASL Clinical Practice Guidelines: Wilson's disease. *J Hepatol* 2012;56:671–85.

Kashi MR, Torres DM, Harrison SA. Current and emerging therapies in nonalcoholic fatty liver disease. *Semin Liver Dis* 2008;28:396–406.

Chronic infection with the hepatitis B (HBV) or C (HCV) virus is the most common cause of chronic liver disease worldwide (Table 7.1). There are an estimated 300 million hepatitis B carriers worldwide and the prevalence of hepatitis B ranges from 0.1 to 20%. The prevalence of hepatitis C also varies geographically and ranges from 0.5 to 15%. Hepatitis is considered chronic when the infection is present for more than 6 months.

Hepatitis B

The prevalence of hepatitis B infection varies worldwide; the highest rates are seen in Asia. The risk factors for acquisition of the virus are discussed in Chapter 1 (page 9).

Chronic hepatitis B is evaluated on the basis of serological profiles, liver function tests and, in some cases, liver histology. A number of patterns of disease are recognized:

- tolerant phase – the virus is replicating actively but there is no evidence of liver damage
- immune clearance phase – immune recognition results in attempts to control viral replication and may cause a clinically recognizable episode of hepatitis (this process can lead to clearance of the virus or to downregulation of viral replication without clearance of the virus)
- persistent replication with evidence of ongoing hepatitis
- intermittent flares in viral replication, which may trigger episodes of hepatitis
- established cirrhosis, with or without evidence of ongoing viral replication.

Serological assessment of chronic hepatitis B can appear complex (Table 7.2). It utilizes two viral proteins – the 'surface' and 'e' antigens (HBsAg and HBeAg) – and their associated antibodies, in addition to hepatitis B DNA. HBsAg is present in all cases of chronic infection. In

TABLE 7.1

Comparison of hepatitis B and hepatitis C viruses

	Hepatitis B virus	Hepatitis C virus
Virus type	DNA	RNA
Prevalence – West	0.1–2%	0.5–1%
– highest	20% China	15% Africa
Worldwide burden	300 million	150 million
Vertical transmission	90%	5%
Sexual transmission	High	Low
Blood-product transmission	Low	Low since 1990–91
Vaccine available	Yes	No
Response to therapy	40–60%	50–85%*
Time to cirrhosis	≥ 5 years	25–30 years
Risk of cirrhosis	20%	25%
Recurrence after liver transplantation	15–20%	99%

*Depending on genotype.

TABLE 7.2

Serological evaluation of hepatitis B

HBsAg	HBsAb	HBeAg	HBeAb	HBV DNA	Status
–	+	–	+	–	Immune
+	–	+	–	+	Replicator
+	–	–	+	–	Non-replicator
+	–	–	+ or –	+	Pre-core mutant
+	–	–	–	–	Seroconverting

+, positive status; –, negative status; HBeAg/Ab, hepatitis B 'e' antigen/antibody; HBsAg/Ab, hepatitis B 'surface' antigen/antibody HBV, hepatitis B virus.

the past, the HBeAg/'e' antibody (HBeAb) status was used to determine whether individuals had active viral replication. Although it remains a reasonable screening test, determination of the replication status by measuring HBV DNA levels in blood is more accurate.

Pre-core mutants of the HBV do not express HBeAg, and infected individuals may not have HBeAb unless they were previously infected with the wild-type virus. In these cases, the viral replication status can only be determined by HBV DNA assay. Seroconversion from HBeAg to HBeAb may cause hepatitis-like symptoms; patients come to clinical attention during this process. Such symptoms can also manifest when both HBeAg and HBeAb are negative. These patients have low HBV DNA levels and will later express HBeAb.

Natural history. Chronic hepatitis develops in 90% of infants and in 5% of adults acquiring the infection. The spectrum of liver disease associated with chronic hepatitis B includes:
• minimal change
• active inflammation with interface hepatitis
• fibrosis
• cirrhosis
• hepatocellular carcinoma (HCC) (usually, but not always, with associated cirrhosis).

Many patients with chronic hepatitis do not develop significant liver disease during their lifetime. The risk of progression to cirrhosis is about 20% over 5 years, and is greater in males than females. Once cirrhosis develops, 85% of patients remain stable for a further 5 years, but the risk of developing symptoms of liver failure increases significantly thereafter. The risk of developing HCC once cirrhosis has developed is 1–2% per year.

Treatment

Pharmacotherapy. Interferon clears the virus in about 40% of cases by increasing immune responsiveness to the virus. The standard dose is 9–10 million units given as a subcutaneous injection three times a week for 4–6 months. Alternatively, 5–6 million units can be administered daily. More recently, peginterferon has been used for the treatment of HBV infection. The potential side effects are significant (Table 7.3).

An expanding number of nucleoside and nucleotide analogs have become available that reliably reduce viral replication and lead to seroconversion to HBeAb in 30–60% of cases with treatment regimens of 3 years or longer. Lamivudine was the first and is extremely well tolerated, but resistance to the drug emerges in a high proportion of cases. Adefovir is slower acting but is ultimately more potent and has a very low resistance rate (about 2% at 1 year). Newer agents like tenofovir, entecavir and telbivudine are increasingly used, either alone or in combinations; they have high resistance thresholds but potentially more side effects.

Liver transplantation is indicated for patients developing liver failure and those found to have small HCCs (typically 1–3 nodules with diameters not exceeding 5 cm on radiological evaluation). Liver decompensation associated with active viral replication has the potential to be dramatically reduced with effective suppression of viral replication, and patients apparently in need of liver transplantation can recover and defer the need for transplantation for many years. The overall burden of hepatitis B on transplant resources is therefore decreasing.

Passive immunoprophylaxis using hepatitis B immunoglobulin, possibly in combination with an oral agent, is successful in preventing reinfection of the liver in 80% or more cases where the HBV DNA is negative at the time of liver transplantation. In the absence of reinfection, the results of liver transplantation for hepatitis B are comparable to those for other patient subgroups.

TABLE 7.3

Side effects of interferon therapy

• Flu-like symptoms on initiation	• Bone-marrow suppression
• Fatigue	• Thyroid dysfunction
• Anorexia and weight loss	• Flares of latent autoimmunity
• Alopecia	• Depression

Hepatitis D (delta) virus is an incomplete virus that can exist only in association with hepatitis B infection. It can be acquired with hepatitis B or can be superimposed on established disease. It seems to lead to more aggressive liver disease, even though, paradoxically, it suppresses the replication of HBV. The incidence of hepatitis D appears to be decreasing. Currently, there are no good treatments available other than interferon.

Hepatitis C

Hepatitis C virus is an RNA virus. The recognized means of acquisition involves contact with blood, and the virus was commonly transmitted via blood products before the introduction of screening for hepatitis C in 1990–91. Intravenous drug use was associated with an infection rate of approximately 70%, and tattooing has resulted in infection with hepatitis C in up to 30% of cases. Sexual and vertical transmission are possible but unusual.

The mode of acquisition in areas of high prevalence is unclear. The prevalence of hepatitis C varies geographically and ranges from 0.5–1% in most Western countries to over 15% in parts of Africa.

Diagnosis. Serological assessment of hepatitis C includes:
- antibody to HCV as the initial screening test
- qualitative polymerase chain reaction (PCR) for HCV RNA as a screen for persistent infection
- quantitative PCR for HCV RNA as a guide to response to therapy
- HCV genotype.

Once HCV antibodies have been detected, the patient should be screened for HCV RNA. Most patients with viremia should have elastography or a liver biopsy, even if the liver function profile is entirely in the normal range, to assess fibrosis and determine if cirrhosis is present. However, the previous pivotal role of the liver biopsy in determining therapy is diminishing with the evolving therapeutic strategies.

Genotypes. There are four main genotypes of HCV.

- Genotype 1 is particularly prevalent in Western countries and in intravenous drug users.
- Genotypes 2 and 3 are most common in northern Europe.
- Genotype 4 is most frequently encountered in Egypt.

The genotype is relevant when assessing the likely response to therapy and in determining the duration of therapy. Hepatitis C is also associated with a phenomenon called quasi-species, which denotes the presence of many strains of the virus within an individual patient.

Natural history. The acute infection is rarely clinically identified and, in most cases, the likely timing of infection can only be determined from an assessment of the risk factors for acquisition of the virus. About 85% of those infected become chronic carriers. Individuals are considered to have spontaneously cleared the virus if tests for HCV RNA are negative on three occasions over a period of at least 2 years.

Infected individuals express a range of liver disease, ranging from mild hepatitis to cirrhosis. The risk of progressing to cirrhosis is 25–30% over a period of up to 30 years. Alcohol consumption accelerates progression to cirrhosis by up to 10 years. Patients over 40 years of age also have more aggressive disease. Once cirrhosis develops, the superimposed risk of developing HCC is in the order of 1–2% per patient-year.

Treatment. The objective of therapy is to get a sustained virological response, which is defined as persistent absence of viremia (qualitative PCR for HCV RNA) more than 6 months after cessation of therapy. This is a rapidly evolving area and the previous standard of care, the combination of pegylated interferon and ribavirin (which has many side effects; see Table 7.3), has recently been improved by the addition of the protease inhibitors telaprevir or boceprevir. Since the introduction of these agents, the rate of sustained virological response in patients with HPV genotype 1 has increased from 40–50% to 70–80%.

Most recently, the first-in-class nucleotide analog inhibitor sofosbuvir has been approved as once-daily oral treatment. Given in combination with ribavirin for adults with HCV genotypes 2 and 3, it is the first all-oral interferon-free therapy. It can also be given in a triple combination with ribavirin and pegylated interferon for treatment-naive patients with HCV genotypes 1 and 4.

These advances are improving overall response rates and reducing the effect of genotype, stage of liver disease and previous responsiveness to interferon therapy on outcome. Clearance of HCV infection in 80% or more of patients will soon be a realistic expectation.

Liver transplantation. Liver disease associated with hepatitis C is now the most common indication for liver transplantation in most countries. Unlike hepatitis B, the burden of hepatitis C on transplant resources is increasing and is not expected to peak for another 10–15 years. The indications for liver transplantation are the same as for hepatitis B. However, unlike hepatitis B, reinfection of the graft is almost inevitable as no immunoprophylaxis is currently available.

Nevertheless, a proportion of patients who are HCV RNA negative at the time of transplantation following antiviral therapy do not develop recurrent infection. Developments in antiviral strategies are expected to be of special benefit to these patients, particularly the significant minority (20–30%) who were at risk of accelerated disease, with cirrhosis developing as early as 3–5 years after transplantation. As a result, the survival rate for hepatitis C was lower than for other indications 8 years and more after liver transplantation. A number of risk factors for accelerated disease have been identified (Table 7.4).

TABLE 7.4

Factors associated with aggressive hepatitis C recurrence after liver transplantation

- Older male recipients
- High viral load before transplant
- Probably genotype 1
- Donor age > 50 years
- Steatotic grafts
- Multiple rejection episodes
- Intensity of immunosuppression

Key points – chronic viral hepatitis

- Hepatitis B and C virus are the most common causes of chronic liver disease and hepatocellular carcinoma worldwide.
- Hepatitis B is preventable with vaccination and is treatable in 40–60% of cases.
- There is no vaccine for hepatitis C, but it is treatable in up to 85% of cases with interferon-based regimens or the new oral therapy sofosbuvir.
- Liver transplantation may be required for end-stage chronic liver disease and small hepatocellular carcinoma.
- Hepatitis C almost invariably recurred after liver transplantation and was problematic, but the availability of additional therapeutic options is likely to change this.

Key references

Bacon BR, Gordon SC, Lawitz E et al. Boceprevir for previously treated chronic HCV genotype 1 infection. *N Eng J Med* 2011;364:1207–17.

Sarrazin C, Hezode C, Zeuzem S, Pawlotsky JM. Antiviral strategies in hepatitis C virus infection. *J Hepatol* 2012;56:S88–100.

Zeuzem S, Andreone P, Pol S et al. Telaprevir for retreatment of HCV infection. *N Eng J Med* 2011;364:2417–28.

Zoulim F, Locarnini S. Management of treatment failure in chronic hepatitis B. *J Hepatol* 2012;56:S112–22.

Cirrhosis is the end result of long-standing injuries to the liver of diverse etiology. Some patients will develop complications of cirrhosis, such as ascites, portal hypertensive bleeding and/or hepatic encephalopathy. These complications may be devastating and portend a poor prognosis.

Ascites

Ascites is the most common complication of cirrhosis and usually heralds a progressive downhill course. Approximately 50% of patients with ascites from cirrhosis will have died after 2 years. Although this chapter deals with ascites caused by cirrhosis, it should be remembered that cirrhosis is not the only cause of fluid accumulation in the abdomen (Table 8.1).

Evaluation. Most patients with cirrhosis will report developing abdominal distension as ascites develops. The patient should be questioned about history or risk factors for liver disease. A history of congestive heart failure, malignancy, pancreatic disease or trauma should be sought. Examination usually reveals a protuberant abdomen with shifting dullness and a fluid thrill. Other stigmata of liver disease

TABLE 8.1

Etiology of ascites

- Liver disease/cirrhosis
- Malignancy
- Heart failure
- Infection (tuberculosis)
- Pancreatitis
- Lymphatic disruption

(palmar erythema, spider nevi, telangiectasia, gynecomastia, etc.) are usually present. Most patients have peripheral edema. Blood tests usually document evidence of liver dysfunction.

Diagnostic paracentesis is mandatory for all patients with new ascites (Table 8.2). Fluid obtained during paracentesis should be sent for measurement of albumin levels, cell count, cytology and culture (ascites should be inoculated into blood culture bottles at the bedside for optimal yield). A peripheral albumin level should be determined. The calculation of the serum–ascites albumin gradient (SAAG) has proved useful for distinguishing ascites associated with portal hypertension from other causes, and is 97% accurate. The SAAG is calculated by subtracting the ascites albumin level from the serum albumin level. If the difference is greater than or equal to 1.1 g/dL, the ascites is a consequence of portal hypertension. Amylase and

TABLE 8.2

Laboratory investigation of ascites

Investigation	Suggestive of
Appearance of ascites	
• Clear/yellow	Cirrhosis, congestive heart failure
• Bloody	Trauma, malignancy
• Milky	Lymphatic disruption
• Cloudy	Infection
SAAG	
• ≥ 1.1 g/dL	Portal hypertension (cirrhosis)
• < 1.1 g/dL	Malignancy
> 250 PMN/mL	Infection
Positive culture	Infection
Amylase	Pancreatitis
Triglycerides	Malignancy
	Disruption of thoracic duct

PMN, polymorphonuclear leukocytes; SAAG, serum–ascites albumin gradient (difference between serum albumin and ascites albumin concentrations).

triglyceride levels may be determined to evaluate ascites due to pancreatic disease or lymphatic disruption, respectively.

Treatment of the underlying liver disease is the optimal treatment of ascites (Table 8.3) but, unfortunately, may not be a practical option. All patients with ascites should restrict their dietary sodium intake to less than 2 g per day. (More severe restrictions are impracticable and may hinder general nutrition.) Fluid restriction to 1.5 liters is advised but may be more stringent in patients with significant hyponatremia.

Diuretics offer relief to many patients. Spironolactone, 100–200 mg daily, combined with furosemide, 40 mg daily, is an effective starting oral regimen. Typical maximum daily doses of spironolactone and furosemide are 400 mg and 160 mg, respectively. Renal function and electrolytes should be monitored frequently and the diuretics adjusted as needed. Rapid diuresis with intravenous diuretics often results in azotemia and electrolyte abnormalities, and should be undertaken with caution.

Large-volume paracentesis (LVP) is a safe and effective technique for the rapid treatment of ascites. Most practitioners remove up to 5–8 liters of fluid at a time, although some perform total paracentesis (removing all ascites at one tap) without ill effects. Most authors recommend the intravenous infusion of albumin after LVP to prevent the systemic hyponatremia and circulatory dysfunction that can follow paracentesis.

TABLE 8.3

Treatment of ascites

- Salt restriction
- Fluid restriction to 1.5 L
- Diuretics: spironolactone, furosemide
- Large-volume paracentesis
- Liver transplantation
- Transjugular intrahepatic portosystemic shunt (TIPS)

Transjugular intrahepatic portosystemic shunts (TIPS) may help patients with ascites refractory to other treatments. TIPS is a radiological procedure in which an expandable metallic stent is tunneled through the hepatic parenchyma to connect the hypertensive portal vasculature to the low-pressure hepatic vein. TIPS is available in many hepatology referral centers.

Liver transplantation should be considered for patients with refractory ascites, provided they are otherwise good candidates (see Chapter 12).

Spontaneous bacterial peritonitis should be suspected in a patient with ascites who is not doing well. The clinical findings associated with spontaneous bacterial peritonitis may be subtle: fever and abdominal pain or tenderness are not common. Vague changes in mental status, electrolyte abnormalities or renal insufficiency may be the only signs and should prompt a diagnostic paracentesis. An ascitic neutrophil count above 250 cells/mm^3 suggests infection and mandates immediate antibiotic treatment, before cultures are available. A third-generation cephalosporin or ampicillin/sulbactam offers good empiric coverage for typical organisms.

Hepatorenal syndrome

Hepatorenal syndrome is a feared complication of cirrhosis, sometimes seen in patients with advanced liver disease and ascites. The kidney responds exuberantly to a relatively low intravascular volume by intense renovascular constriction. Oliguria and azotemia develop. Clinically, the situation appears similar to pre-renal azotemia. Intravenous fluids should be administered to rule out this condition. Midodrine, octreotide and intravenous volume support with albumin may help. Unfortunately, the prognosis is poor but liver transplant may be an option.

Portal hypertensive bleeding

Esophagogastric varices are present in approximately 50% of patients with cirrhosis. Not all patients with varices will bleed, but those who do have a poor prognosis. Despite significant advances in treatment of patients who bleed, mortality remains extraordinarily high. Thus, preventing the first episode of bleeding (primary prevention) is essential for patients at risk.

Primary prevention. Patients with cirrhosis should be screened for varices by endoscopy. If varices of significant size are identified, prophylactic treatment should be started (Table 8.4). The mainstays of prophylactic treatment are non-selective beta-blockers: propranolol (starting dose 20 mg twice daily) or nadolol (40 mg daily) reduce the incidence of bleeding for patients with medium or large esophageal varices. The dosages are increased until the patient's heart rate is 50–60 beats per minute. Endoscopic band ligation may benefit patients who cannot tolerate beta-blockers. Additional research is required before prophylaxis with nitrates can be recommended, and sclerotherapy is not recommended.

Active bleeding. Variceal bleeding is rarely subtle and should be suspected in any patient with gastrointestinal bleeding and a history or evidence of chronic liver disease. The patient often presents in extremis, hypotensive with hematemesis and melena. Resuscitation is the first step in treatment (Table 8.5). Crystalloids usually suffice to stabilize the patient initially, and blood is given to keep the hematocrit in a safe range. Short-term antibiotic prophylaxis with a fluoroquinalone or third-generation cephalosporin has been shown to

TABLE 8.4

Primary prevention of variceal bleeding

- Endoscopy screening of all cirrhotic patients
- Start non-selective beta-blockers in patients with high-risk varices:
  - nadolol, 40 mg daily, or
  - propranolol, 20 mg twice daily
  - titrate dose to keep heart rate at 50–60 beats per minute
- Consider band ligation for those with large varices who cannot tolerate beta-blockers

TABLE 8.5

Treatment of active variceal bleeding

- Rapid resuscitation
- Blood transfusion to keep hemoglobin around 7 g/dL
- Norfloxacin, 400 mg twice daily for 7 days
- Pharmacological agents (use depending on local availability):
  - somatostatin
  - terlipressin
  - octreotide
- Prompt endoscopy with EVL or ES to control bleeding
- Follow-up EVL/ES to obliterate varices – EVL preferred
- TIPS/surgical shunt/balloon tamponade as rescue techniques

ES, endoscopic sclerotherapy; EVL, endoscopic variceal ligation; TIPS, transjugular intrahepatic portosystemic shunt.

reduce the risk of infections that commonly follow variceal bleeding, and improves mortality.

Prompt endoscopy will enable identification of varices and the opportunity to control active bleeding. Several techniques are available.

Endoscopic variceal ligation (EVL) involves the use of small rubber bands to ligate varices. EVL usually controls active bleeding with few complications and is therefore the preferred procedure.

Endoscopic sclerotherapy (ES) involves advancing a thin needle through the endoscope into the varix, and injecting one of several available irritant sclerosants into the varix. Like EVL, ES is effective in controlling bleeding. ES is often easier to perform in patients who are actively bleeding, but is associated with more complications than EVL.

Secondary prevention. Both EVL and ES help to prevent further episodes of bleeding. After control of the first episode of bleeding, 3–5 sessions of EVL or ES are performed to obliterate the varices fully.

Pharmacological control. Much attention has been devoted to the use of pharmacological agents for the control of acute variceal bleeding.

Somatostatin and terlipressin control bleeding in approximately 75% of patients, but neither drug is available in the USA. Octreotide, a long-acting analog of somatostatin with few side effects, has become the agent of choice in the USA, although available evidence regarding efficacy is controversial. The role of octreotide is undefined and it is best regarded as an adjunct to endoscopic techniques.

Transjugular intrahepatic portosystemic shunts (see Figure 2.2) or surgical portal decompressive shunts have a role in patients who have not responded to less dramatic interventions.

Balloon tamponade is effective in controlling bleeding, but an alarming list of associated complications limits its use, and it is currently regarded as a technique of last resort.

Hepatic encephalopathy

Hepatic encephalopathy encompasses a spectrum of neuropsychiatric abnormalities in patients with established liver disease in the absence of other metabolic or structural brain abnormalities. The pathogenesis of the disorder is not fully understood and is an area of active investigation and often heated debate. It is likely that gut-derived ammonia plays some role in the disorder, and theories of endogenous benzodiazepines, false neurotransmitters and brain edema have been postulated.

Clinical presentation and diagnosis. Hepatic encephalopathy can present with a wide range of neuropsychiatric impairment, from subtle alteration in mood, sleep and attention, to stupor and deep coma. Constipation, bleeding, a high-protein diet, electrolyte abnormalities, renal insufficiency and infection may precipitate the syndrome. There are no specific findings on physical examination. Asterixis is frequently elicited, but is not specific for hepatic encephalopathy. Venous ammonia levels are commonly determined in clinical practice, although there is very poor correlation between ammonia levels and clinical presentation.

The diagnosis of hepatic encephalopathy rests upon eliminating other causes for changes in mental status (intoxication, narcosis, subdural hematoma, etc.) in a patient with advanced liver disease.

Treatment of hepatic encephalopathy (Table 8.6) should include correction of precipitating factors. Limiting protein in the diet is reasonable but should be recommended with some caution – many patients with cirrhosis are malnourished, and excessive protein restriction may prevent adequate nourishment. Benzodiazepines and narcotics should be avoided. Renal and electrolyte abnormalities are common in patients with cirrhosis who are taking diuretics, and should be corrected. Infections, particularly spontaneous bacterial peritonitis, should be ruled out.

The mainstay of treatment is the non-absorbable disaccharide lactulose. Lactulose induces catharsis and acidifies the bowel lumen, resulting in the reduction of absorbable neurotoxins (ammonia). Oral lactulose, 15–30 mL one to three times a day, is given to stable patients to produce two or three soft bowel movements per day. Profuse diarrhea may contribute to renal insufficiency and should be avoided. Patients who are acutely encephalopathic often benefit from aggressive dosing until they have bowel movements. Tap-water enemas containing lactulose are used for patients unable to take oral lactulose.

Rifaximin, a non-absorbed oral antibiotic, is effective in controlling hepatic encephalopathy in cirrhotic patients and is usually added at a dose of 550 mg twice daily to therapy with lactulose. A recent multicenter study has indicated that long-term treatment with rifaximin reduces the recurrence of overt hepatic encephalopathy and the rate of hospitalization without any increase in adverse events. In addition, audits in the UK demonstrated significant cost impact by the reduction of hospital admissions and length of stay.

TABLE 8.6

Prevention and treatment of hepatic encephalopathy

- Moderate protein restriction
- Correction of renal and electrolyte abnormalities
- Treat infection
- Discontinue any sedatives/narcotics
- Lactulose orally or by enema
- Consider rifaximin if lactulose fails

Key points – complications of cirrhosis

- Diagnostic paracentesis is mandatory in any patient with new ascites.
- Salt restriction and diuretics are effective in most patients with ascites. Repeated large-volume paracentesis and transjugular intrahepatic portosystemic shunts may be required for refractory cases.
- Patients with cirrhosis should be screened for varices. If these are present, prophylactic treatment with beta-blockers is recommended.
- Acute variceal bleeding is best treated with endoscopic techniques; however, pharmacotherapy also has a limited role.
- Hepatic encephalopathy is a diagnosis of exclusion. Lactulose, rifaximin and correction of precipitating factors are the mainstays of treatment.

Key references

Bajaj JS. The modern management of hepatic encephalopathy. *Aliment Pharmacol Ther* 2010;5:537–47.

Boyer TD, Haskal ZJ; American Association for the Study of Liver Diseases. The role of transjugular intrahepatic portosystemic shunt (TIPS) in the management of portal hypertension: update 2009. *Hepatology* 2010;51:306.

Garcia-Tsao G, Sanyal AJ, Grace ND. Prevention and management of gastroesophageal varices and variceal hemorrhage in cirrhotics. *Hepatology* 2007;46:922–37.

EASL clinical practice guidelines on the management of ascites, spontaneous bacterial peritonitis, and hepatorenal syndrome in cirrhosis. *J Hepatol* 2010;53:397–417.

Runyon BA. Management of patients with ascites due to cirrhosis: an update. *Hepatology* 2009;49:2087–107.

Thomsen TW, Schaffer RW, White B, Setnik GS. Videos in clinical medicine. Paracentesis. *N Engl J Med* 2006;355:e21.

World Gastroenterology Organization. WGO Practice Guideline – Esophageal Varices. June 2008, www. worldgastroenterology.org/treatment-of-esophageal-varices.html

The use of ultrasonography in the investigation of abdominal symptoms and abnormal liver function tests has greatly increased the detection of benign liver lesions (Table 9.1), although the lesions identified are often not relevant to the issue under investigation. Because the detection of focal lesions in the liver can precipitate considerable anxiety until they are characterized as benign, appropriate investigations are warranted and occasionally therapeutic intervention is indicated.

Investigation

The typical investigation pathway after the initial detection is by computed tomography (CT) or MRI. The key questions to be answered about the lesion are:

- is it solid, cystic or both?
- is it vascular or avascular?
- does it contain hepatocytes?
- does it contain Kupffer cells?
- is there a central scar?

TABLE 9.1

Benign focal liver lesions

Common causes	Rare lesions
• Simple cysts	• Nodular regenerative hyperplasia
• Hemangioma	
• Focal nodular hyperplasia	• Pseudolipoma
• Adenoma	• Leiomyoma
	• Lymphangioma
	• Inflammatory pseudotumor
	• Biliary cystadenoma

The characteristics of the more common benign lesions are summarized in Table 9.2.

In uncertain cases, additional information may be obtained from angiography or radionucleotide studies. Lesions that are difficult to classify after radiological evaluation may be further evaluated by biopsy or reassessed radiologically after an interval of 3–6 months. Lesions are considered to be benign if the dimensions and characteristics of the lesion(s) remain constant during that period. It is not uncommon for individuals to have a combination of benign lesions.

Benign liver tumors

Hemangiomas are the most common of all the benign focal lesions and are present in at least 1% of the population. The size is variable but most are solitary, are less than 5 cm in diameter and remain static in size over time (Figure 9.1). Hemangiomas are most commonly found near the capsule of the right lobe. Classic lesions can be diagnosed with a high degree of confidence with any of the radiological techniques, but occasionally complex lesions require extensive investigation. Dynamic scanning using contrast shows a pattern of filling from the edge to the center. The overwhelming

TABLE 9.2

Characteristics of benign liver tumors

Solid	Vascular	Hepatocytes	Kupffer cells	Central scar
Hemangioma				
Complex	Yes	No	No	No
Focal nodular hyperplasia				
Yes	Yes	Yes	Yes	Yes
Adenoma				
Yes	Yes	Yes	No	Maybe
Cyst				
No	No	No	No	No

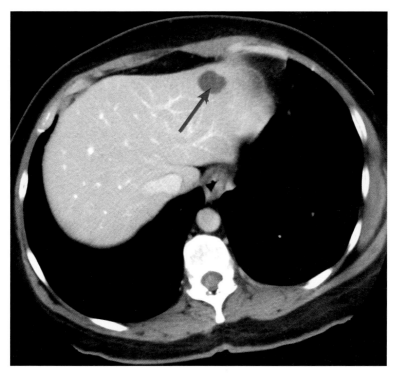

Figure 9.1 CT scan showing a solitary liver hemangioma. Reproduced by Creative Commons licence. CT scan by James Heilman MD.

majority of hemangiomas do not need either extended surveillance or treatment. Occasionally a hemangioma may become so large that intervention is indicated; embolization and surgery are the treatments most commonly utilized.

Focal nodular hyperplasia is the most frequent of the benign solid liver tumors and is most commonly encountered in women during their reproductive years. There is a weak association with exposure to the oral contraceptive pill. The typical lesion is solitary, measures 3–5 cm in diameter and has a characteristic central scar that may be visualized on scanning. About 15% of patients report vague abdominal pain and the remainder are asymptomatic. Unlike adenomas, there is no risk of rupture or malignant transformation and these lesions do not need specific therapy.

Adenomas are rare – about 300 are diagnosed annually in the USA – but are the most clinically relevant of the benign tumors. The development of adenoma is closely linked to use of the oral contraceptive pill in women and androgen therapy in men. Regression after cessation of exposure to the hormonal stimulus may occur but is not consistent. Unlike focal nodular hyperplasia, these lesions have the potential to grow, hemorrhage and rupture. The last two complications may present with severe abdominal pain. Pregnancy increases the risk of rupture, so regular ultrasound surveillance is recommended.

Although rare, malignant transformation is a concern and is one of the reasons to consider resection. Surgical resection is recommended if an adenoma exceeds 10 cm in diameter; however, this is not an option when the lesions are multiple and distributed throughout both lobes of the liver, a condition referred to as adenomatosis.

Cysts

Simple cysts are common and are found in 2.5% of the population. They are most likely to be seen in older women and vary in size from 1 to 20 cm. Most are asymptomatic unless very large or complicated by infection or hemorrhage into the cyst. The appearance on ultrasonography is characteristic as a well-defined echo-free lesion with posterior acoustic enhancement (Figure 9.2). Cysts tend to recur after simple drainage procedures, but may not do so if a sclerosant is injected into the cavity. Defenestration or surgical removal are alternative therapies.

Polycystic liver disease may occur in isolation or in association with polycystic kidney disease. Some cases are associated with congenital hepatic fibrosis. The extent of the cystic change is variable but can lead to near total replacement of the liver parenchyma. Liver transplantation has been performed in cases where the sheer bulk of the liver has become problematic and in cases of venous outflow obstruction (Budd–Chiari syndrome; see Chapter 2). These cysts can also be complicated by hemorrhage and infection.

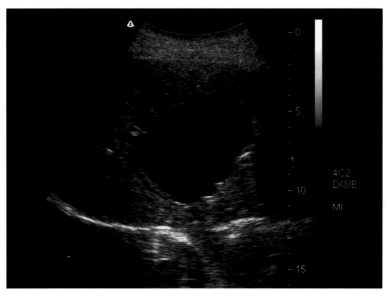

Figure 9.2 Ultrasound scan of a liver cyst, a well-rounded echo-free mass with acoustic enhancement less than 3 cm in diameter.

Choledochal cysts are congenital cystic dilations of the biliary tree. Pain or jaundice are the most common presenting symptoms, typically in young adults. There may be coexisting congenital hepatic fibrosis. Surgical resection may be required.

Infections and abscesses

Pyogenic liver abscesses are discrete pockets of infection within the substance of the liver tissue. Dissemination from a primary source of infection is the most common underlying cause, and portal pyemia complicating intra-abdominal infection such as appendicitis or diverticulitis accounts for a substantial proportion of cases. There are two patterns of abscess: multiple small abscesses distributed throughout the liver, and larger discrete abscesses, which have a predilection for the right lobe. The latter are readily apparent on scanning the liver, but small abscesses may be difficult to detect.

Drainage of larger abscesses is achieved percutaneously or surgically and is the mainstay of treatment. Despite effective drainage, protracted periods of antibiotic therapy are required to eradicate the infection. Antibiotics are the only effective therapy for the smaller, diffuse pattern of infection. Abscesses that develop as a complication of cholangitis may be in direct communication with the biliary tree, and effective drainage may be achieved by endoscopic measures taken to address the cause of the underlying biliary obstruction.

In liver transplant recipients, liver abscesses are either a manifestation of hepatic artery thrombosis or severe cholangitis. The impairment of perfusion that follows hepatic artery occlusion renders antibiotic therapy ineffective, and retransplantation is usually required.

Amebic abscess is caused by *Entamoeba histolytica* and is most common in tropical and subtropical climates. The initial infection may be associated with a diarrheal illness. Discomfort in the right upper quadrant and fever are the main presenting symptoms. The abscess can usually be detected on ultrasonography and is most frequently found in the right lobe. The diagnosis is confirmed by serology. Most cases respond to therapy with metronidazole or tinidazole; drainage or surgery are reserved for difficult cases.

Hydatid disease is caused by infestation with the tapeworm *Echinococcus granulosus*, which resides in dogs but can infect sheep and humans. Symptoms, usually subtle, include fever and abdominal pain. The cysts are detected on ultrasonography or CT and often have characteristic 'daughter cysts' attached to the wall of the dominant cyst. The diagnosis is suggested by positive serology. Percutaneous aspiration of the cysts is not advised. Initial management is with mebendazole or albendazole but many cases will require surgical resection.

Cholangitis is infection in the biliary tree and is usually associated with an obstruction to bile flow (e.g. stone in the common bile duct, benign stricture or malignant disease). The classic triad of symptoms is:
• fever and rigors
• jaundice
• pain in the right upper quadrant.

The treatment consists of antibiotic therapy and, if possible, relief of the underlying obstruction via endoscopic retrograde cholangiopancreatography. Cholecystectomy is indicated in patients with gallstone disease.

Key points – benign liver tumors, cysts, infections and abscesses

- Benign liver lesions are relatively common.
- Most lesions identified are unrelated to the symptoms under investigation.
- Hemangiomas and focal nodular hyperplasia are managed conservatively.
- Adenomas are closely linked to hormone therapy and require surveillance and occasionally surgical resection.

Key reference

Karani J. Benign tumours and cystic diseases of the liver. In: O'Grady JG, Lake JR, Howdle PD, eds. *Comprehensive Clinical Hepatology.* London: Mosby, 2000:ch 24.1, pp 1–13.

Epidemiology and pathogenesis

Hepatocellular carcinoma (hepatoma, HCC) is a malignancy of hepatocytes. HCC is a common cause of mortality in the developing world. Although currently less common in the developed world, the incidence is expected to rise as patients with cirrhosis due to chronic hepatitis C age. Marked geographic variation in incidence is largely due to variation in the risk factors that predispose an individual to the tumor (Table 10.1). Most cases of HCC occur in liver that is already cirrhotic. Thus, patients with advanced viral hepatitis, hemochromatosis or alcoholic liver disease are at risk. Hepatitis B presents a unique risk, as there is evidence that a tumor may develop in the absence of cirrhosis – presumably via direct integration of viral DNA into the host genome.

Clinical presentation

HCC is difficult to diagnose until there is widespread involvement of the liver. Symptoms and changes on physical examination are not specific, and are usually attributed to the underlying liver disorder (Table 10.2). The standard liver biochemical markers are not particularly helpful, although sudden elevations in bilirubin or alkaline phosphatase may suggest obstruction of the biliary tree by a tumor. In the absence of specific clinical findings, most hepatologists suspect

TABLE 10.1

Risk factors for hepatocellular carcinoma

- Cirrhosis of any etiology
- Hepatitis B
- Hepatitis C
- Hemochromatosis
- Aflatoxin exposure

TABLE 10.2

Symptoms and signs of hepatocellular carcinoma

- Abdominal pain
- Hepatomegaly
- Weight loss
- Ascites
- Weakness
- Splenomegaly
- Abdominal swelling
- Wasting
- Jaundice
- Fever

From Kew MC, Hepatic tumors and cysts. In: Feldman M, Friedman LS, Sleisenger MH, eds. *Sleisenger & Fordtran's Gastrointestinal and Liver Disease*, 7th edn. Philadelphia: WB Saunders, 2003:ch 81, p 1578.

HCC when there is a change in the expected clinical course of a patient with otherwise stable liver disease. Paraneoplastic syndromes related to HCC may also give clues to the diagnosis (Table 10.3).

Diagnosis

Because of the non-specific clinical presentation, the diagnosis of HCC is typically made using serum tumor markers, imaging studies and, at times, liver biopsy.

Alpha fetoprotein. Immature (fetal) liver cells synthesize alpha fetoprotein (AFP). Malignant hepatocytes resemble immature hepatocytes, and AFP is an important marker for HCC. A sudden rise in serum AFP or absolute levels greater than 500 ng/mL are highly suggestive of HCC. Lower levels can be seen with any liver disease that provokes hepatocyte regeneration (ongoing hepatitis, cirrhosis). AFP is also produced during pregnancy and by some germ-cell tumors. Unfortunately, not all HCCs produce AFP; 30–40% of patients with

TABLE 10.3

Paraneoplastic syndromes related to hepatocellular carcinoma

- Hypoglycemia
- Hypercalcemia
- Erythrocytosis
- Neuroendocrine syndromes (carcinoid, VIPoma)
- Skin changes (Leser–Trelat sign, pityriasis rotunda, etc.)

VIP, vasoactive intestinal polypeptide.

HCC have normal AFP levels, which considerably limits the usefulness of AFP for screening.

Imaging studies are particularly useful when confirming a diagnosis of HCC. Ultrasonography is inexpensive, safe and convenient. Although widely used, its sensitivity is only about 50%. CT, especially when used with rapid scanning techniques, helps to identify and stage the tumor. It has better sensitivity than ultrasonography, making it particularly useful for detecting small tumors. MRI, angiography and positron emission tomography may each provide additional information. Because of rapidly changing imaging technology and variability in local availability, consultation with a radiologist is strongly recommended.

Biopsy. Many hepatologists believe that suspected HCC lesions (suspected on the basis of imaging characteristics, growth patterns and elevated AFP levels) should not be biopsied for fear that the biopsy may spread the tumor. However, clinicians may be faced with presentations that are less clear, and needle biopsy of the liver is required to confirm the diagnosis.

Screening

Available data do not strongly support the efficacy of screening for HCC. Nevertheless, because there are few symptoms or objective signs of the tumor before it progresses to an incurable stage, and because screening is associated with few risks, many practitioners offer screening to their patients. Patients with established cirrhosis, particularly from viral hepatitis or hemochromatosis, are at the highest risk for HCC. It is therefore reasonable that these candidates be screened, typically with an ultrasound scan and AFP measurement every 6 months. An algorithm for investigating a liver nodule found on hepatic ultrasound is shown in Figure 10.1.

Treatment

Surgery. If tumors are small, there is no evidence of extrahepatic spread and the patient has preserved liver function, surgical resection may be considered. Unfortunately, however, few patients with HCC

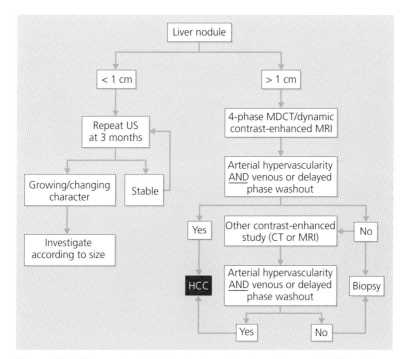

Figure 10.1 Diagnostic algorithm for investigating a liver nodule found on ultrasound (US). Source: American Association for the Study of Liver Diseases. HCC, hepatocellular carcinoma; MDCT, multidetector computed tomography.

have resectable tumors or sufficient hepatic reserve to tolerate a partial hepatectomy, and approximately 50% of tumors will have recurred at 5 years. Liver transplantation may be an option for some patients, provided there is no evidence of extrahepatic spread and the patient is an otherwise good candidate for transplantation (see Chapter 12). The prognosis is best for patients with either a single small tumor (less than 5 cm) or no more than three lesions, each smaller than 3 cm.

Other options. Many patients with HCC are not candidates for liver transplantation or surgical resection. Transarterial chemoembolization (TACE) both embolizes the tumor (to interrupt its blood supply) and infuses chemotherapeutic agents directly into the tumor via the hepatic artery. TACE has been shown to prolong survival but not offer cure. Targeted radiotherapy by arterial infusion of beads has also been used. Ablation techniques may have curative potential for small tumors. Therapy for most patients with HCC is best provided by specialized centers, where patients may be considered for inclusion in randomized controlled trials.

Systemic chemotherapy has a limited role outside of clinical trials. The exception is sorafenib, an oral agent that targets the tumor's blood supply via inhibition of vascular endothelial growth factor. The medication, which is reserved for patients with well-preserved liver function, is generally well tolerated and has modest effects on survival.

Other primary hepatic tumors

Hepatoblastoma is the most common primary hepatic malignancy in children. It usually presents with abdominal swelling, weight loss and failure to thrive, and serum AFP is almost always elevated. Hepatoblastoma is an aggressive tumor and is associated with a poor prognosis; its response to systemic chemotherapy or radiation is inconsistent. If detected in early stages, a well-encapsulated tumor may be surgically resectable. Liver transplantation offers the best potential for long-term survival.

Angiosarcoma is an uncommon malignancy of hepatic mesenchymal cells. Histologically, the tumor is characterized by numerous blood-filled cystic structures lined with malignant endothelial cells. Exposure to arsenic (from insecticides or medications), thorium dioxide and vinyl chloride monomer are well-known risk factors. Like hepatoblastomas, angiosarcomas grow rapidly and are rarely discovered while resectable. Chemotherapy and radiation are usually not helpful, and the prognosis is poor.

Key points – hepatocellular carcinoma

- Hepatocellular carcinoma is a worrisome complication of advanced liver disease.
- Hepatocellular carcinoma often has few specific symptoms or signs.
- Hepatocellular carcinoma should be suspected in patients with an unexpected worsening of liver disease.
- Screening for hepatocellular carcinoma is of unclear utility, but is widely practiced. Regular checking of serum alpha fetoprotein levels and hepatic ultrasound scanning are acceptable.
- Curative treatment by resection or transplantation is an option, but not always possible.
- Radiofrequency ablation, percutaneous ethanol injection, transarterial chemoembolization and systemic chemotherapy are all treatment options.

Key references

Bruix J, Sherman M. AASLD Practice Guideline: Management of hepatocellular carcinoma. An update. *Hepatology* 2011;53:1020–2.

EASL-EORTC clinical practice guidelines: management of hepatocellular carcinoma. *J Hepatol* 2012;56:908–43.

El-Serag HB. Hepatocellular carcinoma. *N Engl J Med* 2011;365:1118–27.

The following aspects should be considered during pregnancy:
- physiological changes
- pregnancy-related liver dysfunction (Figure 11.1)
- management of established chronic liver disease during pregnancy
- coincidental acute liver disease.

Physiological changes

Pregnancy produces cutaneous signs associated with chronic liver disease, including palmar erythema and spider nevi. The majority of the laboratory parameters of liver function remain normal, but:
- alkaline phosphatase increases from the seventh month to term
- serum albumin decreases by up to 20%.

Pregnancy-related liver dysfunction

Hyperemesis gravidarum. Severe vomiting in the first trimester of pregnancy may be associated with abnormal liver function tests, typically a modest elevation in the serum aminotransferases (up to five times the upper limit of normal) and possibly an increased serum

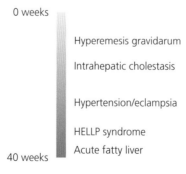

Figure 11.1 Schematic representation of most likely time for development of pregnancy-related liver dysfunction. HELLP, hemolysis, elevated liver enzymes, low platelet count.

bilirubin. The abnormalities resolve with rehydration and control of the vomiting, and no specific therapy is required for the liver.

Cholestasis of pregnancy complicates up to 1% of pregnancies and accounts for 20% of cases of jaundice during pregnancy. It typically presents with itch in the second and third trimesters. Jaundice subsequently develops in association with pale stools and dark urine. The liver function profile shows a marked increase in serum alkaline phosphatase and possibly hyperbilirubinemia. A vitamin-K-responsive coagulopathy may be a manifestation of decreased absorption of fat-soluble vitamins. Management involves control of the pruritus with colestyramine (cholestyramine) or ursodeoxycholic acid. Cholestasis is likely to recur in subsequent pregnancies and with subsequent use of the oral contraceptive pill.

Acute fatty liver of pregnancy presents in the third trimester and is most common in first pregnancies and with a male fetus. The incidence is also increased with twin pregnancies. The presenting symptoms include vomiting, abdominal pain and evidence of fluid retention. Severe cases develop features of acute liver failure (jaundice, hypoglycemia, encephalopathy) in association with evidence of disseminated intravascular coagulation and renal failure.

Acute fatty liver is a mitochondrial cytopathy; the pathogenesis has recently been linked to a genetic deficiency of long-chain 3-hydroxyacyl coenzyme-A dehydrogenase. The liver function profile shows increased serum bilirubin in association with a mild-to-moderate increase in serum aminotransferases. The uric acid level is characteristically elevated. The fatty infiltration of the liver may be apparent on ultrasonography or computed tomography of the liver. Biopsy is rarely required to establish the diagnosis.

Termination of the pregnancy is central to successful management of the condition – clinical improvement is usually apparent within 24 hours of delivery. Severe cases require intravenous fluids, antibiotics and supportive measures for liver and renal insufficiency. The prognosis is good, even in severe cases, and rescue with emergency liver transplantation is only occasionally needed.

Hypertension and eclampsia. Hypertension is a key element of
pre-eclampsia and eclampsia, with additional features including
proteinuria, edema and seizures. The frequency and severity of liver
dysfunction increase with the severity of the syndrome. The dominant
abnormality is in the serum aminotransferases, which may be very
high and in the range associated with acute hepatitis.

The mechanism of injury is fibrinoid necrosis; in severe cases, focal
areas of ischemia are identified on biopsy and radiological assessment.
Acute liver failure, hepatic infarction and rupture are all recognized
complications. Renal failure and thrombocytopenia are other common
features of severe disease. Management involves control of the
hypertension and early termination of the pregnancy. Emergency liver
transplantation may be indicated.

HELLP syndrome is so named for:
• hemolysis
• elevated liver enzymes
• low platelet count.
There is considerable overlap between this syndrome and
hypertension-related liver dysfunction, and management is effectively
the same as for the latter condition (see above).

Pre-existing liver disease
Amenorrhea and infertility are common in patients with cirrhosis.
Conception tends to be a testimony to the degree of preservation of
liver function. Intuitively, one would consider bleeding from varices to
be a significant risk, given the expansion of the intravascular volume
and increasing intra-abdominal pressure. However, this has not been
clearly demonstrated to be the case, and even the stresses of vaginal
delivery are not associated with an increased risk of hemorrhage.

The individual risk of bleeding should be assessed endoscopically
for each woman, and appropriate prophylactic measures instituted. In
most cases, this will mean consideration of propranolol therapy, but
occasionally individuals with mucosal stigmata associated with a
high-risk status may require endoscopic intervention and obliteration
of varices.

Autoimmune hepatitis tends to be fairly quiescent during pregnancy, with flares in disease activity observed in fewer than 10% of cases. However, primary biliary cirrhosis may deteriorate during pregnancy.

Coincidental acute liver disease

Acute viral hepatitis. The clinical courses of hepatitis A and B are unaltered by pregnancy, but mortality is increased with hepatitis E.

Budd–Chiari syndrome. Pregnancy and the postpartum period are times of increased risk for the development of hepatic vein thrombosis in susceptible individuals.

Gallstones. Pregnancy facilitates the development of gallstones, which are found in up to 10% of pregnant women. Biliary obstruction should be managed endoscopically rather than surgically during the pregnancy.

Acute liver failure, unrelated to the pregnancy, may develop after deliberate or accidental paracetamol (acetaminophen) overdose, infection with hepatitis E or other coincidental reasons. Fetal mortality is very high. Maternal care is standard for the condition, and successful liver transplants during pregnancy have been reported.

Adenoma. Surveillance during pregnancy is recommended because of the associated stimulus to growth.

Key points – pregnancy and the liver

- Three classic syndromes of liver dysfunction are associated with late pregnancy: acute fatty liver, hypertension/eclampsia-related dysfunction and HELLP syndrome, but considerable overlap exists between them.
- Cholestasis of pregnancy is a recurrent disorder which is associated with increased fetal mortality.
- Pregnancy is surprisingly well tolerated by women with chronic liver disease.

Key references

Joshi D, James A, Quaglia A et al. Liver disease in pregnancy. *Lancet* 2010;375:594–605.

Su GL, Van Dyke R. Liver disease and pregnancy. In: *Liver Disease: Diagnosis and Management*. Bacon BR, Di Bisceglie AM, eds. Philadelphia: Churchill Livingstone, 2000:344–51.

About 6000 liver transplants are performed annually in both the USA and Europe. After transplant, most patients enjoy long-term survival and dramatic improvements in quality of life. Many patients with advanced liver disease, however, are not candidates for liver transplantation, in part due to the limited supply of donor organs.

Referring physicians should understand the importance of timing the referral for liver transplantation, be familiar with its indications and contraindications and be comfortable with a pretransplantation evaluation.

Indications and contraindications

Liver transplantation may be a viable option for patients with advanced liver disease of almost any etiology. In the USA, the most common indications for transplantation resulting from chronic liver disease are viral hepatitis and alcoholic liver disease (ALD) (Table 12.1). Severe liver disease that has resulted from acute disorders may also require liver transplantation (Table 12.2).

It is important to select candidates who can tolerate the significant physiological, emotional and social stressors that often accompany liver transplantation. An extensive pretransplant evaluation is required to assess the patient's physiological, social and psychiatric reserves (Table 12.3). Accepted contraindications are listed in Table 12.4.

Timing of liver transplantation

Referral criteria for acute and chronic liver disease differ. Acute liver failure is defined as the rapid development of jaundice and encephalopathy in a patient with no history of liver disease. Acute viral hepatitis and drug-induced liver injury are common causes. Criteria have been developed to aid clinician referral of patients with fulminant hepatic failure (Table 12.5). In general, patients with acute liver disease complicated by encephalopathy should be transferred to a liver

TABLE 12.1

Indications for liver transplantation: chronic conditions

Advanced liver disease due to:

- Chronic viral hepatitis
- Alcoholic liver disease
- Autoimmune hepatitis
- Primary biliary cirrhosis
- Primary sclerosing cholangitis
- Hepatocellular carcinoma

Metabolic liver diseases:

- Non-alcoholic fatty liver disease
- Wilson's disease
- Hemochromatosis
- $\alpha 1$ antitrypsin deficiency
- Familial hypercholesterolemia

TABLE 12.2

Indications for liver transplantation: acute liver failure

- Viral hepatitis A, B, etc.
- Seronegative hepatitis or hepatitis of indeterminate cause
- Drug-induced liver disease (paracetamol or idiosyncratic drug reactions)
- Toxin-induced liver disease (e.g. mushroom poisoning)
- Wilson's disease
- Acute fatty liver of pregnancy

transplant center for continued observation and preparation for transplant if needed.

With regard to chronic liver disease, it is best to select patients for liver transplant whose survival would otherwise be dramatically

TABLE 12.3

Pretransplant evaluation

- Routine evaluation of hepatic, renal, thyroid and hematologic function
- Serology for HIV, hepatitis B and C viruses and cytomegalovirus
- Chest radiograph, pulmonary function tests
- Electrocardiogram, echocardiogram and possibly stress test
- Doppler ultrasound evaluation of liver blood vessels
- Contrast computed tomography of abdomen
- Psychosocial and substance abuse evaluation

TABLE 12.4

Contraindications for liver transplant

Absolute
- Active substance/alcohol abuse
- Extrahepatic malignancy
- Ongoing sepsis
- Advanced cardiac or pulmonary disease
- Psychiatric or social difficulties that would interfere with compliance

Relative
- Advanced age
- Severe obesity
- Poor functional status

limited. It must be noted, however, that advanced liver disease itself causes systemic changes that may limit the success of liver transplantation. Thus, the clinician must select patients who are most in need of liver transplant, and are likely to survive the procedure. The

TABLE 12.5

Indications for liver transplant: acute liver disease

Paracetamol (acetaminophen) overdose

- pH < 7.3 (irrespective of grade of encephalopathy)

or

- PT > 100 seconds and serum creatinine > 300 μmol/L (3.4 mg/dL) in patients with grade III or IV encephalopathy

Other patients

- PT > 100 seconds (irrespective of grade of encephalopathy)

or

- Any three of the following variables (irrespective of grade of encephalopathy):
  - age < 10 or > 40 years
  - etiology: non-A non-B hepatitis, halothane hepatitis, idiosyncratic drug reactions
  - duration of jaundice before onset of encephalopathy > 7 days
  - PT > 50 seconds
  - serum bilirubin concentration > 300 μmol/L (17.6 mg/dL)

PT, prothrombin time.

Child's score (Table 12.6) predicts survival for patients with advanced cirrhosis. Patients with a score greater than 7 are likely to benefit from consultation at a liver transplant center. The model for end-stage liver disease (MELD) score predicts survival of patients with cirrhosis using serum bilirubin and creatinine levels and the international normalized ratio (INR). (Calculators are available on the internet, for example at www.mayoclinic.org/medical-professionals/model-end-stage-liver-disease/meld-model-unos-modification). In interpreting the MELD score in hospitalized patients, the 3-month mortality is:

- 71.3% for a MELD score of 40 or more
- 52.6% for 30–39

TABLE 12.6

Determination of Child's score, used to predict the survival of patients with severe cirrhosis

Clinical finding	Points		
	1	2	3
Encephalopathy	None	Grade 1–2	Grade 3–4
Ascites	None	Mild	Moderate
Bilirubin (mg/dL)	< 2	2–3	> 3
(μmol/L)	< 34	34–51	> 51
Albumin (mg/dL)	> 3.5	2.8–3.5	< 2.8
PT (seconds prolonged)	1–3	4–6	> 6

Values in the columns are added for the clinical findings listed
- Child's class A — 5 or 6 points — Patient has well-maintained liver function and excellent expected survival
- Child's class B — 7, 8 or 9 points — Reduced survival
- Child's class C — 10+ points — Very poor prognosis

- 19.6% for 20–29
- 6.0% for 10–19
- 1.9% for a MELD score lower than 9.

Transplant centers use the MELD score to prioritize patients awaiting liver transplant. Acceptable patients should be referred when the MELD rises above 10–12. A similar score for pediatric end-stage liver disease (PELD score) is also available.

Other criteria, including the development of frequent portal hypertensive bleeding, spontaneous bacterial peritonitis or intractable ascites, should prompt referral for liver transplantation. Intractable pruritis associated with cholestasis may also identify potential candidates.

Special concerns

Viral hepatitis. Patients with hepatitis C make up a significant proportion of those undergoing liver transplantation, either because of liver failure or complicating hepatocellular carcinoma. Currently, recurrence of hepatitis C virus (HCV) is almost universal and about one-third of patients get aggressive liver disease. This can lead to the fatal complication of fibrosing cholestatic hepatitis within months, or to cirrhosis within 3–5 years. The survival rates start to become inferior to the other main etiologies at about 8 years after transplantation. Currently, there is a great sense of anticipation that emerging therapies will dramatically improve these outcomes. It has yet to be determined whether the effect will be as great as the equivalent drugs were in patients with hepatitis B.

Hepatitis B was once considered to be particularly aggressive, and its recurrence could result in early graft failure or death. The combination of immunoprophylaxis and the antiretroviral agents has been highly successful in preventing or treating hepatitis B virus (HBV) recurrence. The antiretrovirals also appear to have reduced the need for liver transplantation in these patients because of liver failure, although hepatocellular carcinoma continues to be a common indication.

Alcohol-related cirrhosis. Transplantation for patients with ALD remains controversial. Many clinicians feel that the social and psychological stresses associated with liver transplant would lead to recidivism. These concerns are unconfirmed, however, and it appears that fewer than 20% of well-selected patients return to problem drinking. Survival of patients with ALD following transplantation appears to be comparable to that of transplant patients with non-alcoholic liver disease. Most transplant centers require at least 6 months' abstinence before consideration for liver transplantation.

Living donor liver transplant (LDLT). The limited availability of organs often prevents liver transplantation for candidates who would clearly benefit from the procedure. As an alternative, LDLTs account for about 5% of transplant activity in the USA. This allows an elective operation and access to more grafts in excellent condition. In LDLT, a lobe of the donor's liver (usually from a close relative) is excised and transplanted into the recipient. Because of the liver's rapid regenerative capacity, both organs regenerate to a size appropriate for metabolic activity. LDLT is a technically demanding procedure, but is performed at many centers. Unfortunately, donor morbidity and mortality are realities and potential donors require detailed counseling.

Long-term management of liver transplant recipients

The number of liver transplants being performed annually worldwide is in the region of 15–20 000. It is becoming increasingly likely that medical practitioners will encounter liver transplant recipients on an occasional basis and will need some insight into aspects that differentiate these individuals from their normal patient population. Issues relating to graft function, as well as other complex medical matters, are managed by the transplant centers. However, the recognition and early management of some of these problems will remain in the hands of primary care physicians and non-specialist staff.

Immunosuppression. Liver transplant recipients require long-term immunosuppression, although they tend to be less aggressively immunosuppressed than recipients of other solid organ transplants. Nevertheless, there are issues with:

- immunosuppression per se
- effects of individual immunosuppressive drugs.

Long-term immunosuppression increases the risk of opportunistic infections and malignant disease (Table 12.7). Where indicated, the interval between screenings for malignancy should be reduced (e.g. cervical smears, or colonoscopy in patients with ulcerative colitis, every year rather than every 3 years). Opportunistic infections are relatively uncommon, and the presenting signs are often non-specific. However, it is clear that early recognition is important so that effective therapy can be commenced. This perspective on opportunistic infections is presented on the basis of the possible presenting clinical problems.

TABLE 12.7

Malignant diseases that are more common in liver transplant recipients

- Post-transplant lymphoproliferative disease or lymphoma
- Skin malignancies
- Oropharyngeal carcinoma (especially in alcohol consumers)
- Colonic carcinoma in patients with ulcerative colitis
- Risk-factor-associated malignancy (e.g. lung cancer in smokers)

Cough and other respiratory symptoms are a common presentation; most cases are caused by familiar community infections. Vaccination against influenza is recommended for liver transplant recipients and should reduce the incidence of influenza in these patients. Antibiotic therapy is widely used to prevent or treat superimposed bacterial bronchitis, which is a common sequel to viral respiratory tract infections. Opportunistic infections should be considered if:
- symptoms do not resolve within the expected time period
- shortness of breath develops, particularly if this is disproportionate to findings on chest radiograph
- associated findings occur (e.g. lymphadenopathy).

Cytomegalovirus, *Pneumocystis carinii*, aspergillosis and mycobacterial infections are the main opportunistic infections that present with respiratory symptoms.
- Infection with cytomegalovirus tends to occur within the first year of transplantation and is typically associated with a very high fever.
- *Pneumocystis carinii* presents with a dry cough and shortness of breath.
- Mycobacterial infections may present with hemoptysis or have associated lymphadenopathy.

Diarrhea is another frequent problem and is usually the result of drug toxicity or common infections. The latter are generally well tolerated, and management is as standard for immunocompetent individuals. However, diarrhea may also be the presentation of an opportunistic infection. *Clostridium difficile* is common in the early post-transplant period when exposure to broad-spectrum antibiotics is high. Reactivation of the infection can occur in the community, and a stool sample should be screened in patients known to have had previous infection. Cytomegalovirus can cause gastroenteritis, and this should be considered in patients with high fevers, abdominal pain or rectal bleeding.

Lymphadenopathy. Lymphoma or post-transplant lymphoproliferative disease (PTLD) must be considered in any patient with unexplained lymphadenopathy. This is the most common non-cutaneous malignant disease after liver transplantation and can present at any time. The risk of developing PTLD correlates roughly with the cumulative intensity of immunosuppression, but all patients should be considered at risk. Suspected cases should be referred immediately to specialist centers. Mycobacterial infections, both typical and atypical, should be considered if there are associated respiratory symptoms and when the distribution is predominantly in the cervical region.

Pyrexia of unknown origin. Unexplained fevers, especially in association with non-specific systemic symptoms such as anorexia and weight loss, may be indicative of PTLD.

Immunosuppressive drugs. The majority of liver transplant recipients are maintained on an immunosuppression regimen based on calcineurin inhibition with either tacrolimus or ciclosporin (cyclosporine). These may be used in combination with other drugs to increase potency or, more commonly, to reduce the toxicity of individual drugs. Other agents for maintenance immunosuppression include prednisone, azathioprine, or mycophenolate and sirolimus or everolimus. Transplant centers are usually responsible for monitoring drug dosing.

Side effects. All of the immunosuppressive drugs have potential side effects (Table 12.8). However, some of these are sufficiently common in the context of liver transplantation (e.g. headache and diarrhea) that extensive investigation is unnecessary. Other potential side effects require careful prospective monitoring, with adjustments to the

TABLE 12.8

Side effects of long-term immunosuppressive regimens

General
- Malignant disease
- Opportunistic infections

Common and possibly considered tolerable
- Tremor
- Headache
- Diarrhea
- Hirsutism
- Gingival hyperplasia
- Alopecia

Common but requiring intervention
- Hypertension
- Diabetes mellitus
- Gout
- Weight gain/obesity

Requiring specific monitoring
- Impaired renal function
- Hyperlipidemia
- Osteoporosis

immunosuppressive regimen if necessary. A typical example is the nephrotoxicity associated with long-term use of calcineurin inhibitors – up to 25% of liver transplant recipients have chronic renal failure 10 years after transplantation. This is being addressed by reducing reliance on calcineurin inhibitors. Hypertension is another common side effect and it, together with diabetes mellitus, may contribute to the recognized progressive deterioration in renal function.

Drug interactions. The potential for drug interactions is great, but in patients taking ciclosporin or tacrolimus the following two points are of particular importance.

- Avoid non-steroidal anti-inflammatory drugs and any antibiotic ending in '-mycin' (e.g. clarithromycin) because of the threat of renal failure (even with short-term use).
- Among herbal remedies, St John's wort should be avoided.

Disease recurrence. Many liver diseases have the potential to recur after liver transplantation (Table 12.9). The liver transplant center will normally screen for recurrent disease, but some diseases may first become apparent to the primary care physician (e.g. ALD), whereas others may be co-managed in the community (e.g. hepatitis C).

Vaccinations. Only live or attenuated vaccines are contraindicated.

Contraception and reproduction. Sexual function in men and fertility in premenopausal women is usually restored after liver transplantation. Intrauterine contraceptive devices may cause infection and should be used with care. Hormonal contraception is

TABLE 12.9

Diseases that commonly recur after liver transplantation

Common, may threaten graft/patient survival

- Hepatitis C (near-universal, variable progression)
- Hepatitis B (15% despite prophylaxis)
- Excessive alcohol consumption (15%)
- Hepatocellular carcinoma (15–20%)
- Other malignant diseases

Lower impact on graft function

- Alcohol consumption
- Autoimmune hepatitis
- Primary biliary cirrhosis
- Primary sclerosing cholangitis
- Budd–Chiari syndrome

contraindicated in patients with prothrombotic disorders, particularly Budd–Chiari syndrome. Pregnancy is generally well tolerated but transplant patients have a higher incidence of some complications (e.g. hypertension, low birth weight).

Dietary restrictions pertinent to chronic liver disease (e.g. salt or protein restriction) no longer apply. Restriction of calorie intake is important in the 20–25% of patients with accelerated weight gain or obesity. Dietary adjustments are needed in patients with diabetes mellitus, hyperlipidemia or hypertension. Some foods are contraindicated because of the risk of infection (e.g. paté, uncooked shellfish, unpasteurized cheeses).

Key points – liver transplantation

- Liver transplantation is effective for a wide range of liver diseases.
- Thorough assessment is mandatory and must cover physiological, social and psychiatric comorbidity.
- Many diseases recur after transplantation, but with variable consequences.
- Careful attention to the complications of immunosuppression is of great importance; possible opportunistic infections, drug interactions and side effects can occur.
- Limitations to lifestyle after transplantation are remarkably few.

Key references

Lucey MR, Terrault N, Ojo L et al. Long-term management of the successful adult liver transplant: 2012 practice guideline by the American Association for the Study of Liver Diseases and the American Society of Transplantation. *Liver Transpl* 2013;19:3–26.

Murray KF, Carithers RL. AASLD Practice Guidelines: Evaluation of the Patient for Liver Transplantation. *Hepatology* 2005;41:1–26.

Wiesner R, Edwards E, Freeman R et al. Model for end-stage liver disease (MELD) and allocation of donor livers. *Gastroenterology* 2003;124:91–6.

Useful resources

USA
American Association for the
Study of Liver Diseases
Tel: +1 703 299 9766
aasld@aasld.org
www.aasld.org

American Gastroenterological
Association
Tel: +1 301 654 2055
member@gastro.org
www.gastro.org

American Liver Foundation
Helpline: 1 800 465 4837
www.liverfoundation.org

National Cancer Institute
Tel: +1 800 422 6237
www.cancer.gov/cancertopics/
types/liver

National Digestive Diseases
Information Clearinghouse
www.digestive.niddk.nih.gov/
ddiseases/a-z.asp

UK
British Association for the Study
of the Liver
Tel: +44 (0)1543 442154
admin@basl.org.uk
www.basl.org.uk

British Liver Trust
Info line: 0800 652 7330
Tel: +44 (0)1425 481320
info@britishlivertrust.org.uk
www.britishlivertrust.org.uk

British Society of
Gastroenterology
Tel: +44 (0)20 7935 3150
www.bsg.org.uk

Cancer Research UK
Speak to a nurse: 0808 800 4040
Tel: 0300 123 1022
www.cancerresearchuk.org/
about-cancer/type/liver-cancer

King's College Hospital Liver
Transplants
www.kch.nhs.uk/service/cancer/
treatments-for-cancer/transplants

Macmillan Cancer Support
Helpline: 0808 800 00 00
www.macmillan.org.uk

International
Australian Liver Foundation
Tel: 0417 785679
www.liver.org.au

European Association for the Study of the Liver
Tel: +41 (0)22 807 03 60
easloffice@easloffice.eu
www.easl.eu

European Liver Patients Association
contact@elpa-info.org
www.elpa-info.org

Gastroenterological Society of Australia
Toll-free: 1300 766 176
gesa@gesa.org.au
www.gesa.org.au

Other resources
AUDIT – Alcohol Use Disorders Identification Test. Guidelines for Use in Primary Care: whqlibdoc.who.int/hq/2001/WHO_MSD_MSB_01.6a.pdf

CAGE questionnaire: www.integration.samhsa.gov/clinical-practice/sbirt/CAGE_questionaire.pdf

Maddrey's Discriminant Function for Alcoholic Hepatitis: www.mdcalc.com/maddreys-discriminant-function-for-alcoholic-hepatitis

MELD calculator: optn.transplant.hrsa.gov/converge/resources/MeldPeldCalculator.asp?index=98

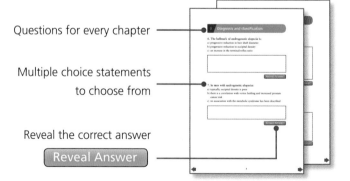

FastTest

You've read the book ... now test yourself with key questions from the authors

Questions for every chapter

Multiple choice statements to choose from

Reveal the correct answer

Reveal Answer

FREE at fastfacts.com

- Go to: www.fastfacts.com/fast-facts/Liver-Disorders-2nd-edn
- Click on the *FastTest* to open the interactive PDF

Index

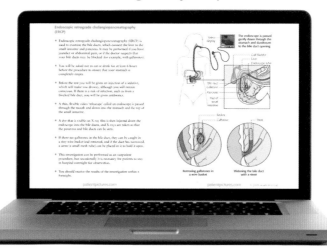

Your Aha! Moment?

A moment of sudden realization, inspiration, insight recognition or comprehension

Did you have one when reading this text? That is our aim at *Fast Facts*, but we don't want you to keep it to yourself. Share your Aha! Moments and read others at:

www.fastfacts.com/fast-facts/Liver-Disorders-2nd-edn

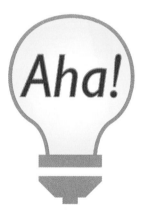

And if you found this book useful, please consider sharing it with your colleagues or students. A book recommendation from someone you work with is often the best kind, so send this title on a journey around your clinic or department and help us on our mission **to promote health, effectively.**

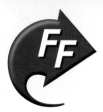

Fast Facts – the ultimate medical handbook series covers over 60 topics, including:

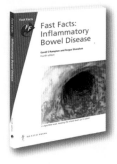

Fast Facts: Inflammatory Bowel Disease

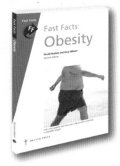

Fast Facts: Obesity

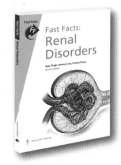

Fast Facts: Renal Disorders

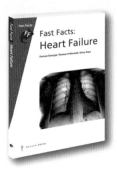

Fast Facts: Heart Failure

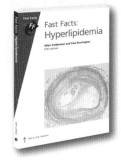

Fast Facts: Hyperlipidemia

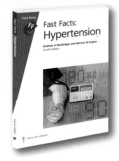

Fast Facts: Hypertension

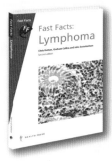

Fast Facts: Lymphoma

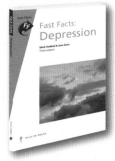

Fast Facts: Depression

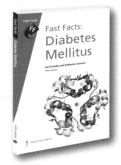

Fast Facts: Diabetes Mellitus

fastfacts.com